Who Is Taking Care of My Mother

Who Is Taking Care of My Mother

Carrie Caine

Copyright © 2011 by Carrie Caine.

Library of Congress Control Number:	2010919143
ISBN: Hardcover	978-1-4568-4068-6
Softcover	978-1-4568-4067-9
eBook	978-1-4568-4069-3

All rights reserved. No part of this book may be reproduced or transmitted in any form or by any means, electronic or mechanical, including photocopying, recording, or by any information storage and retrieval system, without permission in writing from the copyright owner.

Any people depicted in stock imagery provided by Thinkstock are models, and such images are being used for illustrative purposes only.
Certain stock imagery © Thinkstock.

Print information available on the last page.

Rev. date: 05/03/2017

To order additional copies of this book, contact:
Xlibris
1-888-795-4274
www.Xlibris.com
Orders@Xlibris.com

OUTLINE

I. Overview 9
   To bring some awareness about caregivers/caregiving and how I went about
II. Introduction 13
   What motivated me to write this book
III. Chapter One 17
   I am a Caregiver
     How and why I became a caregiver
IV. Chapter two 23
   A. Details about Words
      1. Respect
      2. Dignity
      3. Abuse
      4. Neglect
   B. Example of each word
V. Chapter three 29
   The working Care Giver
   A. Interview with other Caregivers
   B. Money is a common problem
   C. List of do's and don'ts for caregiver working in different types of care facilities.
   D. List of other problems you may find
VI. Chapter Four 53
   Language Game
   A. Changes in Words and Phrases
   B. Example of Writing
   C. Why Language Affects Caregivers

VII. Chapter Five 62
The Formula for Caregivers, three specials qualities.
Desire + Education + Training = Experience = Success
   A. All about the three Special Qualities
   B. Why they are so important
   C. The benefit they bring
      1. Experience
      2. Success

VIII. Chapter Six 74
The care of an individual from a Professional Level/Point of View
   A. The facility, or an individual gives you instructions.
   B. A list of people you might care for in a care facility or someone home.
   C. A list of health problems they may have

IX. Chapter Seven 78
The care of an individual from a Personal Level/Point of View
   1. You're responsible for:
      A. Physical care
      B. Personal Care
      C. Emotional Care
      D. Health Care
      E. Social Care
      F. Making decisions
      G. Safety
   1. Feeling and Emotion
   2. Guilty

X. Chapter Eight 81
Looking for a Care Facility
   A. Define the different types of adult care facility
   B. Some reasons it may be hard to find a care facility
      1. Money
      2. Time

        C.   Examples
            1.   Personal
            2.   None personal
        D.   Knowing what question to ask, things to look for, and things do

XI.   Chapter Nine 92
      Looking for a Caregiver or Needing a Caregiver
        A.   Use an agency
        B.   On your own
        C.   Don't lose control
            1.   Activity involved
            2.   Representative/Advocate
        E.   Two stories
        F.   Use of a caregiver's application
        G.   Application

XII.   Chapter Ten 106
      Stress and Burnout
        A.   Caregiver should watch out
        B.   How it affected me
        C.   Information is important

XIII. Chapter Eleven 113
      Training Program
        A.   The benefit of having one
        B.   Facility can develop one per their needs
        C.   A basic Training Program, Outline

XIV. Conclusion 120
        A.   Changes I hope this book bring to caregiver all over
        B.   My last thoughts what a good caregiver looks like
        C.   How being a caregiver has tested me?

OVERVIEW

I have compiled a lot of information in this book to share with you. I do not pretend to have all the answers, but I think I can bring some awareness to a very important subject, called caregiver/caregiving. I am a Caregiver; I will share some information from my education, training, and experience, personal and Professional. Caregivers are very important people in society today. At some point, half of the population may need a caregiver and the other half may become caregivers. Caregivers/caregiving has two categories, personal and professional. We will look at both categories from personal care, physical care, health care, social care, and emotional care. We will look at some very important words caregivers should know in detail. We will explore the working caregivers, which is also the professional caregivers. We will see that caregiving looks different when you go to work in a care facility. I will share some interviews from other caregivers about their experience, and problems. I will show you how money seems to be a common problem. There is a list of do's, and don'ts when working with different people. I will discuss how, many problems in care facilities come from the lack of education, and training of employees. I will show you how your written words can affect a working caregiver. We will look at some examples of words, phrases, and words changes. I will talk about the language game that goes on in care facilities.

The next two chapter, will focus on the care of an individual from a professional level/ point of view, and a personal level/ point of view. Most of the time when you are a caregiver for pay it is professional and you should do what people tell you to do. You must remember your feelings and emotions are not important. The feeling, and emotions of the person you are caring for is important. We will look at their needs and who determined those needs. Some facilities provide some of the care, the caregiver does not have to do it all. These care facilities have their own departments or a person to do certain things like, laundry, activities, passing out medication, and transportation. In other care facilities, the caregiver is responsible for doing those things. Most of the time when you are the caregiver for a family member or loved one it is personal. Your feeling, and emotion are very important, many decisions comes from them. You're responsible for every aspect of the person's life. We will also explore how your feeling make you feel obligated to take care of someone. We will discuss the qualities and mindset, I think caregivers should process if they are going to be a successful caregiver. We will discuss the formula in detail (Desire + Education + Training = Experience =Success).

There may come a time in a person's life he or she may have to find a care facility or a caregiver. Finding a care facility or a caregiver is not an easy task. It can cause you a lot of pain and distress. You should know something before seeking a care facility or a caregiver. We will define some of the different types of adult care facilities. We will explore how you make your decision about a care facility. I will show you, how your decisions could have a negative impact. I will share my personal experience. People should know what questions to ask, what to look for and what they need to do. We will explore how to find a caregiver, and who pays the caregiver. Your responsibility to the caregiver. We'll find out what happens when you lose control over the situation. Be actively involved in the care of your family member, be an advocate. We will look at a story about a man named John. We will view a caregiver application, and the power of the application. We will look at stress and burnout, they are two very real factors when you are a caregiver. We will explore why they are very important. I will talk a little about how stress and burnout affected me.

In the last chapter, we will talk about the important of a training program. I will cover some of the basic training of new and old employees who work in care facilities as a caregiver. I will cover some of the training I think I should have had in the beginning of my career as a caregiver. We will look at some ways it could help facilities that do not have a training program in place or improve the one they do have. We will look at an outline of a basic training program. In conclusion, I will share my hope for this book and my last thoughts about what a good caregiver looks like. Being a caregiver has tested me in many ways.

INTRODUCTION

I was inspired to write this book because of my personal and professional experience as a caregiver. I was hearing and seeing some of the things that happened to people who were under the care of others. Every time I heard something on the news about an elderly person, child, or person with disability being abuse or neglected by their caregiver or in a care facility, it just made me sick. My first thought, what is wrong with people? People decide to be a caregiver and take care of others; I wonder, do they know what that means? I just did not understand why these things were happening so much. Was it all the caregiver's fault, or was it the care facility, or both? I decided to study myself first. I remember situations I found myself in when I started working as a professional caregiver. My first title, was not a caregiver; I was a nurse's aide. I have had several different titles over the years. When I first worked in a nursing home, I remember the feelings I had about the people I was taking care of. You take care of people you do not know. You rely on the people in the facility to train you, or show you where to find the information. This is where some care facilities fall short. The nursing home gave me a quick orientation, and training about the job. After the training, they left me on my own. There were times I did not know what to do or who to ask. I felt they hired me, and said, "Learn as you go". I decided to learn, and kept on learning. I had to start with, what I knew, and what I thought I knew. I made many mistakes. I found out there is a wright way and a wrong way to take care of someone in a care facility. No one told me about the politics I would have to work under, and deal with.

Care facilities must do certain things to keep their license, so they write their own policies, and procedures. There are rules and regulations from the government they must follow. Government rules and regulations change constantly in a care facility. You might be doing something wrong and do not know it. The meaning of words can also change. Your written words or documentation is very important when working as a caregiver in a care facility. Some words can imply abuse depending on how you use them. Sometimes care facilities get so caught up with government expectation they lose sight of their clients/resident wellbeing. The caregiver cannot lose sight of their clients/resident's wellbeing, that is another reason a good training program is important. If the nursing home had a better training program, I would not have been so confused. Some care facilities do not have any type of orientation, or training program. They let you follow, or shadow another staff, you watch what he/she does one to five days and that is your training. When you are trained that way, you only get half of what you will need to do your job. Many of my mistakes as a working caregiver had to do with my writing/documentation. Care facilities want to make sure everything looks and sounds good on paper. More than one person reads your writing/documentation. You could have three different interpretations about what you wrote, and that is the language game.

What happened when you do not use a care facility, but you still need a caregiver. You could go through several people before you find the right caregiver. You always can get an agency to find someone for you, but will you be satisfied. Finding a caregiver, yourself may give you some satisfaction, because you get to interview the person. How would you know if you are asking the right questions, and going about it the right way?

This can be a very stressful task. Developing a strategy, be in control and know what kind of person you're looking for.

By the time, I became my parent's caregiver I thought I could do it with ease. I had several years of experience by then. Boy was I wrong. I was faced with being a caregiver on a personal level. Being the caregiver for my parents was the hardest job I have ever had. I could not forget those feeling and emotion I was having. I had to be the caregiver for people who used to care for me. They were my loved ones. You may think when you are the caregiver for a family member it is the same as a loved one. You may learn it is not.

I AM A CAREGIVER

As I mentioned I am a caregiver. I have had several different titles or positions as a caregiver. I do not care what title or position the care facilities pined on me, I worked as a caregiver. I want to talk about how I became a caregiver. I was sixteen, and my school selected me to work in a summer program. I was excited about working, because it meant I would have my own money. I went to work in a nursing home; I knew I was going to hate that job, because I knew nothing about old people. That is what we called elderly people then. I did not care about old people one way, or another even though, I had a grandfather at that time. I didn't really know him, I knew he was my grandfather, and I loved him, but I did not know the person. I knew one of my grandmothers for about twelve years, then she died; I never knew the other. So, at sixteen, all I knew about old people and people who needed help was nothing. I remember hearing stories like old people smelled funny. Old people do not know anything. Old people were crazy, mean, and grouchy. Some people said you could not understand what they said, and they had diseases. There were other stories also. I though some of the stories were true because my mother was always helping my grandfather, so I thought he did not know much.

I went to work in this nursing home with negative thoughts. I intended to hate that job the whole summer. I was going to do my work and not talk to anybody, because something was wrong with everybody, and I did not want to catch anything. One day I went into a woman's room, she was blind. I said a quick hello. I had to help her go to the bathroom clean her up and dress her. I also had to fix her bed. I was not saying anything to the woman. She began to talk to me, she said, "How are you doing?" At first, I said nothing, because I thought she was talking to herself. I remember, old people talk to them self all the time. The woman said it again, and I looked at her, and asked "are you talking to me?" The woman said, "yes is anyone else in the room?" I said "no ma'am". She started asking me questions, like what was my name, how long had I work there. I was shocked because they were normal question. She talked to me while I was in the room, and all of it made sense. When I left her room I said "bye", she said "bye" also. I shook my head, not sure what had happened. Did I really carry on a conversation with this person or not? So, the next room I went into, I spoke first, and that person started to talk also. It went on like that all day. The people were carrying on a conversation with me. I was not really listening to the conversation; I was surprise they made sense. The next day, I started all over again. This time, I wanted to hear the conversation. Some people talk about their life before they came to live in the nursing home. I met people who were normal. I met some retired teachers, a retired pharmacist, and I even met a man who told me he was a mortician. I was not sure what a mortician did at that time. That man was happy to tell me all about his job. I met all types of interesting people. I stopped focusing on the work I was doing. I started learning things from those people, not things about themselves, but things about people in general, and life. I began to realize they were people who started out in this world just like me. They were intelligent people who had done a lot in their life. They were full of life and had so much to tell. I began to absorb things from them. They taught me things school was not going to teach me. I discovered that those people deserve the the highest respect. I learned things about myself, like, I did not mind helping people, and most of the people I was helping where know different from me, just older. They had experience some of the same things in their younger days, I was experiencing right then. I was beginning to like the people, not the work. I was sixteen, and I was thinking about someone else beside myself. I changed that summer, but I would not realize it until later in my life.

    I thought, I would become many things, but never a caregiver, not once, because I remember working in that nursing home. Even though I liked the people at that nursing home. I would hear some of the regular workers talking to the old people and some of the things they were saying weren't nice. Since I felt the way I did about old people, it did not bother me. Before that summer was over it had started to bother me. That summer stayed with me, I became very sensitive to older people feeling. I became more aware of what came out of my mouth. I started noticing my grandfather. By the next school year, I was looking at my older teachers differently. I think I became more respectful. I began to feel like only older people could teach me, because they had been where I had to go. I started listening to things my grandfather would say; I was evening listening to my parents more. I started listening to older people who had something they wanted to tell me. I still did not realize all the changes that had come over me. One day, a friend, and I were walking home from school, and I stopped at her house for a while. I found myself in the kitchen with my friend's mother, having a conversation, and enjoying it. My friend wanted to know, who I came to see, her or her mother; I laughed, and I realized I rather talk to her mother. It became easy for me to develop a relationship with older people. They were so eager to teach and show me things. It was as if it made them happy to know a young person was interested in listening to them.

    I finished high school and decided I wanted to sit behind a desk doing clerical work. I attended a career center to learn how to be a clerk typist. There was a young girl in my class; she was in a wheelchair. I noticed her right away. At first I thought it was because people with physical disabilities stood out, but then I noticed the way she acted and the way people treated her. People made special efforts to move out of her way, always ask her if she needed help. I could see it bothered her a little. I started talking to her; I learned she had some of the same issues the people in that nursing home had. She felt people were not treating her like a human being. She did not like people making a lot of fuss over her. She said she could do a whole lot of things by herself. She explained; most people just saw her disability, not her ability. She told me she drove herself to school. Not everybody can do that. She had a wonderful sense of humor. She was not an old person. She was not much older than I was. She had a disability that prevented her from doing some things and she needed help doing other things. We did not become best friend, or anything like that, but I learned older people were not the only ones with disability.

I finished the course, got my certificate, went to work at a desk, and was not happy. I did not feel like I was doing anything worthwhile. I was not meeting people. I was not really helping anyone. I remembered, when I was helping people, and felt good; was the summer I worked in that nursing home. At the end, I enjoyed working with the people, and that made the work tolerable. I decided, I wanted to work in a field where I could help people, and make a different in their life, young, and old with, or without disabilities. The problem was, there was a lot of things I could do. I could be a nurse, I did not want to be a nurse. I wanted to do some of the things a nurse did, but not function solely as a nurse. I could be a social worker, but I did not think I could put my personal touch in my work. There were so many boundaries in being a social worker also. Those are just two ways I could help people, and there were a lot more.

I met someone who told me, she was a Human Services Worker. She explained some of the things she did. I realized it was a broad field, but it would allow me to learn something about different areas of helping people (older people, disabled people, people with mental illness, and intellectual disabilities) and still be in a profession. As a Human Services Worker, I could work in different care facilities. As a Human Services Worker, I could learn a lot about other things that go along with helping people. I wanted to understand people emotions. Why people do some of the things they do. I wanted to understand the family relationship, and things to look for during the aging process. I wanted to learn communication skills. As I thought about it anybody could be a Human Services Worker, doctors, lawyers, teachers, even a custodian worker. Think about it! What is the major role of those people? It is to help people. I also found out a Human Services Worker is a caregiver.

Therefore, I went to school for Human Service. I took many psychology classes. Those classes help me a great deal in the way I relate people. Those classes taught me how to recognize behavior changes. I learned when to listen and how to listen. I learned how feelings and emotion can affect the care a person receives. I was learning about guidelines, code of ethics, and all sort of other things, I would need when I go to work as a Human Service worker. I Decided, I would focus on the caregiving said of Human Services. I liked how I felt when I worked in that nursing home. I also realize I did not mind the work I was doing. School also gave me a chance to practice as a caregiver in different types of care facilities. Some of the care facilities were nursing homes, adult homes, hospitals, residential homes. I received my Associate Degree in Human Services. I also had a chance to get my certificate in Adult Home administration, because I wanted to learn something about the administrators said of care facilities. Over the years, I have attended many conferences, convention, seminars, workshops, and joined organization, all related to caregivers, and caregiving.

Some things school could not teach me. One very important lesson, people are different no matter what their situation or circumstances are. You cannot put people in a box. You cannot say everybody in the box is the same in every way. You cannot take care of them the same way. Some time you cannot dress two people the same way, for example, one may want his socks on first, and one may want his paints on first, they are the same age living in the same nursing home, so you do not just get them dress. School tends to put people in a box. I had to learn how to care for people on a one-to-one. Every elderly person, or persons with disabilities did not need the same care, or in the same way. That became part of my training.

When I became my parent's caregiver, the knowledge I received from school helped me to recognize their decline. I start thinking about what I might have to do early regarding their care. I knew what resources I would need. School could not help me with the physical care or my feelings and emotions. I had to deal with all of that on my own. I had to rely on my experience and training I received as a professional caregiver.

So, when I think back on my journey to become a caregiver. I remember this was not what I thought I would be doing, then I remember (Psalms 32: 8)

> "I will instruct you and teach you in the way which you shall go: I will guide you with my eyes" K J V

That verse said it all; I am a Caregiver.

Respect, Dignity, Abuse, and Neglect

The first thing I learned as a caregiver was the definition of four words. You will see and use these words repeatedly throughout your career and life. Those words are Respect, Dignity, Abuse, and Neglect. Let us see why these words are so important. Most of us learned the word "respect" growing up. Respect to me means anything nice, or showing courtesy to someone because of who and what, they are (a human being). I have seen the word just vanish when you find yourself caring for someone other than a family member, or a love one, and sometimes even when it is a family member. Some people fell it is hard to respect someone who is cursing at you, and hitting you, or just plain mean. As a caregiver, you must respect the people you take care of no matter what. See the person as an individual, like you want to be seen. You already know a caregiver can be anybody that cares for someone. That includes a doctor.

Everyone wants to trust a doctor, because he/she supposed to make you well, and you pay him/her for the services. I was surprised when I met a very disrespectful doctor. I went into his office with pain in my leg, and shoulder. He did not ask me my name. He did not even look at me, when he came into the room. I did have an appointment, but when he finally looked at me, he said he was busy so he could only deal with one of my problems, and I had to come back for the other. He asked me which one hurt worse. I could not answer. I told him I would make another appointment, and I left. All caregivers can learn more about respect. Some people have a hard time respecting people they may not like or know. Sometimes when you respect a person, it can change how that person look at you.

Dignity is another word I think goes along with respect. Dignity to me means, something you do, or something someone does for you that make you feel good about yourself, an act that does not make you feel ashamed, or bad. There are many ways people do not give respect, or dignity to others. You are not giving a person their respect or dignity when you treat them like they are not human or they do not have feelings. You are not giving respect or dignity to a person, when you speak bad or use foul language against them. When you are taking care of someone, and you do not do your best, you are not giving them their respect, or dignity. You would be very surprised to see how happy you can make people when you give them their dignity, and respect. When I am working with a person with disabilities, or an elderly person, I try to imagine how, I want be treated under the same circumstances. I want people to treat me with dignity and respect even if I did not know it.

Here is some situation, where I failed to show an individual dignity or respect. When I was in school I had to do some practicum work. My first practicum work was at a nursing home; I was still learning, but I knew a little about nursing homes from my experience in high school. However, I was just starting to understand the words dignity, and respect, and how it relates to caregiving. From my high school experience, I know older people could talk. At the nursing home, I would walk down the hall speaking to the residents, some of them would be sitting in their room with the door open, and some would be walking down the hall. One day, I walked down the hall like always, speaking. I walked by a room, and the door was stretched wide open. I began to speak; I saw a woman sitting in a chair with nothing on. She had nothing to cover herself with. I remember feeling embarrassed for her, but I just walked by. I saw the person who was supposed to be taking care of the woman. She was on the telephone, talking, laughing, and shaken her head. I realize what I should have done, was given the woman something to cover herself with, and shut the door. The other thing I should have done was report the person. I remember the woman head hanging down; she could have felt embarrassed also. Her dignity, and respect was taken from her, and she could not do anything about it.

I did my second practicum work at another care facility, it was my first day. A staff was showing me around. I noticed another staff coming out of a room. I heard the staff say to the person in the room, "see you later, Bob." The staff was smiling when she said it, so I thought it was real. I went back to introduce myself to Bob. I knocked on the door, and went in, I said, "Hi, Mr. Bob, I'm new." That is all I got out of my mouth before Bob started cursing, and swearing at me. All I remember hearing, something about the name Bob before I flew out the door. I thought to myself, this is not for me! I went to another staff to tell her what happened to me; she wanted to know who did that. I told her it was Mr. Bob, and she wanted to know who Mr. Bob was. I took her to his room, and she laughed she told me his name was not Bob. I said, that was the name I heard someone call him. She explained, staff calls him that when they want to make him mad. I was upset with myself! I did not check, to see what the man's name was. I should have just knocked on the door, told him my name, and let him tell me his name. I disrespected the man, by calling him another name other than his own.

By the time, I got to my last practicum work, I thought I knew something. To my surprise, I still did not know anything. I was assign to help a woman get dressed for the day. I thought she was unable to help herself. You would have thought; I would have learned by now. Always ask! I pick out a dress I though was pretty. It was red and white. I put the dress on her, and she asked me, why I put that "shit" on her, I replied, "What?" she repeated herself. I apologized, and asked her what she wanted to put on? She had no problem picking her own dress out. Again, I failed to ask questions; I did not find anything out about the women before I went into her room. I just went to her room, to put clothes on her.

There was one more situation regarding dignity and respect, I was not, prepared for. My assignment was an eighty-seven-year-old Caucasian woman in a wheelchair. I was helping her put on her knee-high stockings. The stockings kept sliding down her leg, and I kept pulling them up. So, I finally decided to get her another pair, and they were fine. The woman looked at me, and said, "I am glad you took those dam stockings off, because you had me looking like a nigger". I do not know, if she said that for me or not. I do know she looked at me, and did not say a word when I enter her room. I was shocked, and offended; you can say I get mad. I walked out of the room and left her. I was supposed to take her to breakfast. I said I was not going to take her anywhere. I do not think elderly people talk like that especially to people who were taking care of them. I was still learning, and that was a real revelation. I had never experienced that, even when I was younger working in that nursing homes. The biggest mistake I made with this woman, I took what she said personally. I was an employee, and that is how I should have acted. I should have respected the woman, and done my job anyway. As a caregiver, you will run into all kinds of people, and there may be some racial, and other discrimination issue.

I had another racial experience in the same care facility. I like to go into the residents' room, and talk to them. This woman was still very active in her community; she was a painter, and could paint beautiful pictures. She can have intelligent conversation with you. I enjoyed talking to her. I never paid too much attention to her remarks about different race of people;

I just thought she was making conversation. One day, she asked me to pick up a greeting card for her. I told her I would walk with her to the gift shop to get a card. She implied they did not carry the type of card she wanted. It was a religion card, not her religion, but someone else. She went on talking about, how the facility did not deal with certain types of people. I just told her, I would pick up the card. I got the card, and took it to her. She still wanted to talk about the card. I nicely change the subject. So, then she pulls out this beautiful outfit. She told me she brought it to celebrate Black history month. I realize she really wanted to talk about this; so, I let her talk. She told me, she was going to put it on, and walk around the facility. I replied that was nice. She said everyone will be mad with her, but she did not care. Therefore, I had to ask what she meant. She just came right out, and said it, "You know they don't like black people here." I knew all that talking was for me. She just would not stop talking, then she said, I liked black people, and she had black friends. She started laughing. I told her I had to go. I did not go back to see the woman anymore. One day I saw her in the hall, and she asked me, if she offended me in any way. I asked her, if she thought she had offended me, and walked away. I started taking everything personal. I started bringing my personal feelings to work. I am not saying she was right, what she said about that facility, but I felt she did have a problem with me. After that experience, I started having a lot of problem with dignity, and respect around there. I became very unhappy at that facility. I realized I needed to learn so much more about dignity, and respect, so my personal feeling would not interfere with my work.

Now, let look at the words "abuse" and "neglect". I think abuse means doing something physically, or mentally to a person with the intent to cause harm, or unhappiness. Neglect to me means not providing care, shelter, food, clothing, and any other support for a person under your care or supervision. In many situations; I found out, proper training, and education could have prevented some of the abuse, and neglect in care facilities, and with people under the care of a caregivers. When you work as a caregiver in a care facility, you should always be watchful to make sure you do not abuse or neglect anyone. Abusing or neglecting someone can carry a jail sentences. That is why it is so important to understand what abuse, and neglect mean, and why a person should have a lot of training in this area. Like I mention earlier laws are continuously changing in this area. For example, some of the things people used to do to their children/child, and adults are abusive, and neglectful now. In addition, what you may think is not abuse, or neglect, the law may say otherwise. It is sad to say, but some care facilities hire people, and do not review anything about abuse, or neglect. I guess they think everybody knows about that. Most people, think they know what abuse, and neglect means. If you are not sure, you know what they mean, as a caregiver you should find out. We do have an organization that deals with this on a high level. You could be banned, or lose your license, if you hold on. Most of the time a charge like abuse, or neglect can stop a person from working in the field of caregiving, and remember you can go to jail.

You will need to know as much as possible about these four words, if you are going to be a successful caregiver. Your action, and response to these words can make or break you. I look at these words in this way: If I do not respect myself, how can I respect others? If I do not have any dignity myself, how can I give someone else his or her dignity? If I abuse, and neglect myself, how would I treat others? It means a lot to an elderly person, or a person with disabilities, when you give them their respect, and dignity, and you do not abuse or neglect them. Elderly people, and people with disabilities are easy target for abuse, and neglect. It is a concern for all caregivers and everybody.

THE WORKING CAREGIVER

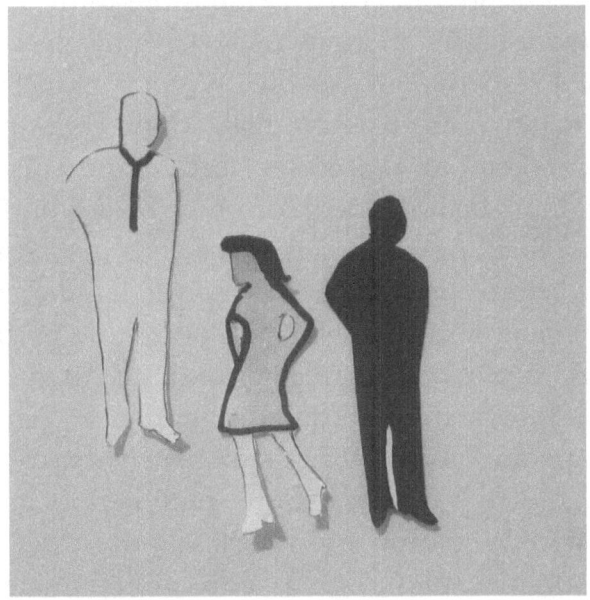

I looked up the word "Caregiver" in the dictionary. One of the definitions implies a person who gives direct care to someone. That definition did not give the word justice. So, after reading all those definition, I came up with my own version. Caregiver is someone who cares for someone else's needs by giving him or her help or support in an area or areas of their life where they need it. It can be help or support with personal care, physical care, social care, emotional care, health care, it also can be legal, or financial care. Let's look at these types of care from a caregiver point of view, and what you might be doing. The first care is personal care; it is helping, or assisting an individual with all their needs like taken a shower or bath, Oral hygiene, dressing, grooming, changing depends or diapers. Physical care; you may have to pull, left, push a wheelchair, clean, feed someone or cut up food. You might provide transportation as well. Social care, you provide support to an individual to help him/her become independent in areas of their life, like cooking, cleaning doing laundry, getting involve with the outside world. Emotional care, helping the individual develop close, and meaningful relationship; getting his/her family, and friends involve in the person life. When it comes to Health Care, you might preform some basic duties; like passing out medication, taken blood pressure, and temperature. You may have to monitor the individual for other health problems, and report it to a doctor or someone else who is in charge. Most of the time a license professional caregiver handles the health care part. Legal, and financial care is handle by the facility, and a license professional caregiver also. Just to give you some background information on the word caregiver/caregiving.

A lot of people do not think caregiver/caregiving jobs are important, and that is why, I think some people do not see it as a profession. When you go to work as a caregiver in some of these care facilities, they give you a different job titles. Some of the titles I am familiar with, are Nurse Aide, DSP, Residential Counsel, Training Assistant, Direct care, and CNA's. I am sure there are some more titles people have had. The title does not change the work you do. I'm here to let you know caregiver/caregiving are very important, and it is also a profession no matter what people want you to think. I found out that the word caregiver/ caregiving was first used in 1966, but the word care in association with caregiver/caregiving can be traced before the 12th century. Another word that was use before the word caregiver/caregiving, was the word caretaker, which was first used in 1801. This information is very important, because it lets you know caregivers, and caregiving has been around a long time.

When you finish reading this book, I think you will feel caregivers are important, because they hold someone's life in their hands, not just the physical stuff. As a caregiver, you might have a lot to do with the person's state of mind. You may be surprised at the effect, you could have on a person life, when you are taking care of them. You could be the only friend that person has. You may be the only person he/she responds to. You may be the only person he/ she goes anywhere with. You may be the only person he/she feels safe around. A caregiver, wear many hats: a teacher, trainer, protector, counsel, driver, maid, the person who listen, healer, fixer, and a role model. You may even be that person's eyes, and ears. Some jobs a caregiver has might turn your stomach, if you have a weak one, and some jobs have safety concerns, you must protect yourself. There is a lot of information out there, telling you how to care for certain people, like the elderly, those with dementia, children, and the disabled. I found out early, it is not the care that is the biggest problem; It is who is given the care. Most caregivers have not read all that information out there, about how to care for people. When you get a job as a caregiver, some on the job training should take place. People who are hire as caregivers should have the right attitude. We will talk about that later.

In this book, we will focus on caregiver/ caregiving for adults, or adult care with, and without disabilities. Sometimes you hear things in the news about abuse, and neglect in nursing homes, adult homes, and other care facilities. We know the building, and the furniture is not doing it; it is the people who work there. Some care facilities failed to do good reference checks on their new employees. It is very important to check reference before you heir someone. Some care facilities do not do that, some of them put the person to work, and find out there is a problem later. Some facilities say they check reference, but I know from my own experience that is not always so. Did you know a lot of these care facilities, only require a caregiver, to have a high school diploma, and you must pass a background check? That is all good if the care facility has a good training program. You know a person background can change over a period, just something to keep in mind. I cannot tell you how many people, I have worked with, and wonder how they got the job. How long a person has worked as a caregiver is important. You will read something about that later. Caregivers are needed all over, because it is not enough good caregivers around. It is very important to know who is taking care of your loved one.

I have spent a lot of time working as a Caregiver for adults, both as a career, and in my personal life. I have learned a lot and have seen a lot. When I first started out, every interview I went on for a caregiver's job gave me information about the physical care, and the personal care, I would be doing. I found out later, after I got the job, their where things they forgot to tell me. They tend to leave out things like, you may have to deal with complaining family members. You may not have all the things you need to do your job. You may have to cut corners, which prevents you from doing your job right. You may have to put up with a lot of negative personalities. You might have to learn techniques on how to protect yourself, and others from harm. You may be working with people who has behavior problem. You might have to working alone. You may be working with people who have more than one problem. You may have to learn CPR, and basic first aid, you may have to conduct safety drills. You may have to pass out medication, you might have to take a test for that. You might have to provide transportation. You may have to deal with some racial issues, and sometimes those are the hardest things to deal with. Then, there are those discrimination issues care facility might try to hide. You know the ones that say you cannot advance in this business! Those are some of the things you may not see in your job description.

Remember, there are different types of care facilities, so you may not be doing the same things in them all.

Some care facilities go beyond personal, and physical care; you can see that by some of the things you might have to do. Some of these things are very good, and they give you good experience, and training; it would help to know a lot of these things up front, before you accept the job. Believe me for some people it would make a different. I have talked to people who said they did not know what they were getting into when they took a caregiver's job. I think care facilities should give as much information as they can to new employees about the job. You may get rid of the people that weren't going to work out anyway. When you don't give all the information about a caregiving job, the job sounds much easier than it is, and anybody thinks he/she can do.

People become caregivers for many reasons, and a lot of the time, it doesn't have anything to do with helping people. Sometimes they just need a job, and they believing it's easy. Some people think they can make a lot of money as a caregiver. A lot of people think they can always find a job as a caregiver. Is that true? I don't know, but I do know there is a great need. You already know you don't have to have a caregiving background to become a caregiver. Remember, you can become a caregiver for a family member, your next-door neighbor, or anybody. When you become a working caregiver in a care facility, you take on different roles, and different responsibility. You have rules, regulations, and laws you must follow. These rules, regulations and laws can break or make a care facility, and the working caregiver. When working as a caregiver in these facility, you should make yourself aware of all the rules, regulations, and laws.

I keep talking about care facilities, let's be clear about the types of care facilities I am referring to. These type of care facilities take care of the elderly with, and without disabilities, people with mental illness, or other mental health problems.

People with developmental disabilities of any kind. The people who live in these types of care facilities are unable to live by themselves, and are unable, or need assistance to care for themselves in one or more areas of their life. Then you have people who end up in these care facility, because of a fall or accident they might go home at some point. Also, most of these types of care facilities are staff 24 hours a day. The other thing about working in these care facility, you may have 4 to 8 people you are responsible for during the day. You will read more about the different types of care facilities in another chapter.

I have observed so many things working as a caregiver. I have seen some bad things, and some good things. I wanted to know how other working caregivers felt, so I started asking questions. I spoke to people who said they hated their job, but the pay was decent, and they could live off it. Some people said, they didn't get paid enough money to do this kind of work. Some people said that was all they knew how to do, and some people said they just needed a job. People said caregiving was easy work, because no one is looking over your shoulder. Some people felt they would always have a job as a caregiver. So, I went deeper. I wanted to know more about the people who said they hated their job. Hate is a strong word, and it can lead to abuse, and neglect. I wanted to know what they hated about the job, because that's important. I started with myself first, I thought about the summer I worked in that nursing home, and why I hated it at first. I ask myself many times, what was I doing there, because I did not like working with old people. Then I realized I did not know anything about old people, and I did not have any training in that type of work. I did not know anything about helping people. Those were the reason I hated the job, but I thought just like other people, I was getting decent money. That was the only incentive I had at sixteen. Some people hated the type of work they had to do to get the money, and they did not like helping people. They hated the way their clothes smelled when they went home. Some of them hated, they had to respect each person they were taking care of. Some caregivers, felt the clients/resident did not respect them, so they did not want to respect the clients/residents. There are individuals some caregivers refused to help or assist; they let their personal feeling get in. That is a recipe for abuse, and neglect. Some of the people I was talking to had been trained, or had a degree. I figure, when you get a degree, this is the kind of work you want to do, how wrong was I? I asked some of the people, who said you will always have a job as a caregiver. They explained; people were living longer, and getting sicker, and the country will always need people to take care of them. They also said you did not have to know what you were doing. They felt most care facilities were all about making money. They said the main key to getting a caregiving job was to say, "I like to helping people."

Then, you have those working caregivers who likes to do private duty work. Those are the people who get a job as a personal caregiver in someone's home. You do have some families who do not want to put their love one in care facilities, so, they hire a caregiver. I had a chance to interview some private duty caregivers also. these are some of the things they said. One person said if you work for a family a longtime, and the person you were taking care of dies; the family may give you money. Some people said they knew someone that happen to. Another person said it was very laid back, because you are taking care of one person. There were people who said they loved the people they were taking care of. Some people said everything was cut and dry, you did not have to do anything extra. Most people go through an agency to get their private duty caregiver, that will be discuss later in this book.

I continue with my interviews. Some people, said they borrow money, clothes, and other items from the individual they were taking care of. They said no one checked behind staff. They did not do any inventory of the individual's things. They could sneak stuff out, and put it back, no one knew anything. A person told me they took some jewelry from one of their individual, and pawned it, because they needed the money to pay a bill. The individual got the jewelry back, and no one ever knew. I thought how careless the facility was. Another person said "I eat the food off the individual's plate.

A lot of care facilities are in regular house, run like a regular home. These care facilities are set up in regular communities. These types of care facilities are called residential home, or group home. A lot of the individuals who lives in these types of care facilities have Intellectual disabilities. or some other type of developmental disabilities. These houses have everything a regular home has including a washer and dryer. I think these types of care facilities are a recipe for house abuse, and position abuse. Staff has an opportunity to take care of their own needs, and wants. Some people said they bring their clothes from home, and wash and dry them. They would take items like, toilet paper, paper towels, and detergent from the house. By the way, if you don't know, that is stealing. Some caregivers said, the things that frustrated them the most, about these care facilities, were the double standing stuff that goes on. For example, the individuals living in these type care facilities have rights, just like all of us. They have the right to say no, but as the caregiver working there, it is your reasonability to encourage the individual to say yes to some things. You deal with things you think means something to the individual, and things you feel the individual needs. It makes you question wither the individual has all their rights; the line gets confusing in these types of care facilities. You play a lot with words.

Believe me, there are good caregivers out here. These are some positive things people said about being a caregiver. One person said, she likes what she does. She like working with older people, they make her day. One person said, she went into this field, because of a loved one. Some people felt they would be good at taking care of people. Some people wanted to learn, so they could start their own facility. Some people said, they saw how bad older people were treated in some of these care facilities, and they wanted to change that. People said, they like to talk, and get advice from older people. One person said, she felt good, when she saw the look on a resident face, when she thanked her for giving her a bath. She's said the resident thanked her several times. Most of the people living in care facilities are so grateful for the people who take care of them. Another person said it was easy to build a trusting relationship with them. I don't know about that one. I think it takes a little time to gain someone's trust. One person said she was thankful for the experience, because it helped her, in her personal life. These things may not sound like a lot, but they can cover many area of a person life.

I know it's hard to believe some of the things people said, but there are worst thing people did not say. I know this, because of my own experience. People had no problem talking to me. I told them I might write about it someday. They said they did not care, because I was not using their name. Some of the people I interviewed, have gotten out of the caregiving field, and unfortunate some of them moved to other facilities. The bad things, I heard did bother me, but I knew how real they were.

Out of all the negative, and positive things people said about being a caregiver, both group had one thing in common. They felt they do not get paid enough money to do, or put up with some of the things they had to. I can agree with them, because how can you put a price on the care of a human being? How can someone else treat your loved one, as well as you can, when they do not know them? How much money is enough, to get physically attacked by someone you are taking care of, and that person has emotional problem.? How much money is enough, to be verbal abused by a family member of someone you are taking care of; and having to hear nothing you do is right? How much money is enough, when you work by yourself, and you take care of people at a ratio of one caregiver to six individuals? Don't forget everyone should be ready at the same time. How much money is enough, to have to deal with racial, or other discrimination issues every day? How much money is enough, to be disrespected on a regular basis? Believe me; you will never make enough money. You may become satisfied, I don't know. Since money plays a big role in this field, let's look at it more closely.

Let's say you were making $15.00 an hour; that is good money. After you make that for a little while, and you have to clean people with feces all over themselves every day, you start to feel like $15.00 an hour is not enough money. You get a $5.00 raise, and now you're making $20.00 an hour. You're still doing the same things. For a while, you're satisfied with that $5.00 raise. That doesn't last long; you get tired of going home smelling like urine, feces, and someone spits on you. Again, you start to think a $5.00 raise is not enough. You see how this could go on, and on. The essential point, you're still doing the same things every day, and you may have to put up with some other, unpleasant things, no matter what they pay you. Some people move to different care facility, because they pay more money. In a short time, you find negative things there also, the work is the same, and you might be doing more. People job hop a lot in this profession, always looking for more money, and less work. I encourage you before you move to another care facility, because they pay more money, ask yourself some questions.

1. Am I doing this just for the money?
2. Do the people respect me (clients/residents?
3. Do I liked the place where I work?
4. Can I grow here?
5. Does the care facility respect my knowledge?
6. Do I get along with my peers/coworkers?
7. Do I get time off when I need it?
8. Have I had any personnel problems?
9. Do I have a problem doing my job?
10. Is my supervisor always on my back?

11. Am I tired of doing this type of work?
12. Have you done something that may cause you to get firer?
13. Am I the real problem?

Those are just a few questions you should ask yourself, before moving to another care facility. Sometimes you can have so many other problems working in care facilities, money is your least concern, (you're facing an abuse charge, have violated someone confidentiality, you failed to report a case of abuse or neglect to the proper authority). When you come to those points, you should get yourself another profession.

Before I move on, I think I should mention two other important issue a working caregiver should be aware of. The first one is confidentiality. You know the world is big on confidentiality today. Basic that means a person who works for a company, or the company cannot give out any information about someone without his/her consent or permission. There is some exception. A care facility takes that even further. You cannot talk about anyone you'll taking care of, in their present, or around other people even, if you think they do not know what you are saying. You cannot reveal any information to a family member without permission, unless the person you are taking care of, is a minor. Confidentially is worth learning more about. Here is two example of confidentially.

John is a 22-year-old male that was admitted into the hospital, a family member came to see him. The family member stopped at the nurses' station. She wanted to know what was wrong with John. The nurse informed the family member, she needed to talk to John. The family member got upset, stating she was John's mother, and she was entitled to all his information. The nurse explained, she did not see her name anywhere, and John was an adult, they could not give her any information without his permission. They could give information if he was a minor or unable to give his permission.

Next example: Jan was in a restaurant with a friend. She was telling her friend about an individual she was taking care of. She was revealing personal information about the person. There were people setting all around them. Jan violated confidentiality and she disrespected the person she was taking care of. You never know who, knows who, and a fellow employee could have been sitting in one of the table around her. You should never talk in public about people.

The next issue, you are a mandated reporter. If you witness someone violating an individual right or abusing, and neglecting an individual, or even if you suspect a person is being abuse, or neglected you must report it to the proper authority. There are consequences if you do not report it. Here is an example of a mandated reporter.

CeCe and Jan works at a care facility. CeCe witness Jan hitting, Mr. Doe, because he did not do what she told him to do. CeCe did not report it. The next day, the supervisor noticed Mr. Doe face was swollen. Mr. Doe told what happened to him, and who was present, CeCe and Jan was terminated, CeCe was terminated, because she failed to report the incident. She did not follow the procedure of a mandated reporter.

While talking to people, they gave me a list of some problems they faced, while working in some of these care facilities. I can surely relate to some of them, because I have faced some of the same problems during my career. I am going to share this list with you, and then I will give you an example.

1. No respect or lack of respect from your employer or supervisor. (your supervisor talks down to you. They do not think your job is important. They do not respect your judgment, until it is too late, even then they don't acknowledge it).
2. The living-in- a barn feeling. (Employer and supervisor act like you don't know anything about neatness or cleanness).

3. Questioning your documentation. (Staff writers down something he/ she notices about an individual, supervisor ignores it, and does not act on it until he/ she noticed the same thing).
4. Lack of promotion, because a lot of caregivers don't hold a degree, some employer feels they cannot do anything else. It doesn't matter how long he/ she has been doing the job).
5. Lack of rights, (There is a sheet posted in each facility, telling employees about their rights and labor laws. Some employers found loophole to do employees out of them when something goes wrong or they have their own interpretation).
6. Lack of staff, (you don't have enough staff to do your job; you have to let some things go, no matter how important they are).
7. Lack of ideals, (You give supervisor an ideal and he/she ignores it or doesn't feel you know what you are talking about. Three months down the line, he/she use your idea and call it theirs).
8. Staff morale, employer and supervisor do not appreciate staff for anything extra they do without pay. (Like when you work an extra hour to help staff out just, because you want to or when you're flexible to suit the company's need, you get no credit for anything).
9. Personal feelings, supervisor, and other staff let their personal feelings interfere with their job. It doesn't matter the person is a good worker. It is something about him/ her I don't like).
10. Training/lack of training, (staff do not know what they need to know about the job. Staff is not aware of new things, or changes that has taken place).
11. You think you know me, (employer, and supervisor think, because you work as a caregiver you have no ambition or

goals for your life. They feel you have an unproductive life, so they try to hold you back).
12. It's all about the supervisor, (you do whatever I tell you to do no matter what).
13. Safety, (when you work in a care facility for a while, you know the place. You notice something that is unsafe for the individuals you're caring for, you report your concerns. Your concerns are ignored and something happen. Staff are sometimes made the scapegoat and accused of neglect or abuse).
14. The thin line, (The rules and regulations say one thing, but what you can do is something else).

You know there is two sides to everything, and sometimes there is more than two side. The second said to the employee's view of the problems are the supervisors view of the problems. I had an opportunity to interview some supervisors also. They gave me a list of some of their problems.

1. Unprofessional, (when employees have a problem, they come to talk, they talk at you not to you. They are loud and they fuss at you. They come to work looking any kind of way, no respect).
2. They complain about everything even, if it is a government policy or company policy (nothing is right).
3. Always late for work, (getting an attitude when you mention it).
4. Not showing up for work (History of calling out).
5. Not a team worker, (don't try to help their coworkers, don't care how they leave the workplace for the next person).
6. Easy to get offended, (you can't say anything to them).
7. Lazy, (When it is work they don't want to do, or they say, that is not my job).
8. Make excuses, (that did not happen, because).

9. Treating the work place like your home (not realizing this is a job).
10. Stealing, (They think if they take something small it is not stealing pencil, Paper, paper clip etc.).
11. Sneaky, (think no one knows what is going on)
12. Personal feelings, (incorporating your personal lifestyle and feelings within the job, doing things your way).
13. Making assumptions, (feeling like you're being personally attacked).
14. Conflict, (asking others to cover for them, causing confusion).
15. Incompliance with rules and regulations (not keeping up with training).
16. Not realizing there's a bigger picture, (blame the supervisor for everything).

A lot of employees don't realize, there is a lot of politics in running a care facility. If you don't believe that, try to open one up. Most employees think, what they see on the surface is all it takes to running a care facility. Some decision a care facility make, they have too, so they can stay in business. The two lists above do not cover all the issues of employees or supervisors, don't forget there are different types of care facilities. Regulations are code the government has set for care facilities and employees to follow. A lot of the time, facilities fail to do the things that are needed to keep the facility up to code. Sometime employees get caught doing their job without the proper equipment, material, or enough staff. The facility management knows all of this, but they hope nothing happens. Unfortunately, a lot of the time, when something bad happen in a care facility, the blame can fall on an employee. Some of the problem I have seen, management could have prevented them. One of the reason for the problems, half of the staff do not have proper training, so they do things wrong. Some of the time the quality of work is not up to code. Sometime care facilities have money problems. Staff is stressed out from been over worked no relief time. Do all your home work if your dream is to open a care facility. You already know you need to hire staff. The longer I work with people, the more I learn. The more I talk to people, the more I learn.

When I worked with different people, I notice a lot of do's, and don'ts. These do's. and don'ts have helped me throughout my career, with other people, and on my job. This list of do's, and don'ts, I pick up, when I worked with the elderly, those with dementia, and Alzheimer's. Now, this is the list I keep in mind when I am in the presence of an elderly person.

1. Show respect for the individual, and yourself.
2. Give him\her their dignity.
3. Make the individual feels safe, and secure.
4. Don't talk about an individual in their presence (like they are not there).
5. Do not embarrass anyone.
6. Be alert anything can happen.
7. Do not allow your personal feelings to interfere with the way you care of an individual.
8. Do not force your way of doing things on anyone.
9. Do not get involved, in a personal battle with the person you are taking care of.
10. Make sure you give good grooming and hygiene care.
11. If there is something you don't know about an individual, always ask.
12. Do not handle an individual in a rough manner.
13. Make sure you don't bruise or hurt anyone while you are taking care of their needs.
14. Do not make an individual feel inferior to you.
15. Do not assume an individual does not know what he\she wants.
16. Honor an individual's wishes, if possible.

17. Always try to make an individual as comfortable as possible.
18. Always called an individual by his/her name, or the name he/she prefers.
19. Do not assume you know what is hurting an individual, because you do not see it (pain is not always seen).
20. If an individual can go to the bathroom, let them. Do not put a dapper or depend on the person, because it is easy for you.
21. Do not take anything from an individual, even if you feel the person has given it to you. The person may not be aware of what he/she is doing.
22. Do not force, or threaten an individual to do anything he/she does not want to do.
23. Do not give unnecessary medication, because it makes your shift easy. (sleeping pills, etc.)
24. Do not make an individual's bathroom yours.
25. Do not turn an individual's television on, because you want to sneak back and watch it.
26. Always think first before you react. (Control yourself)
27. Do not eat the food off an individual's plates.
28. Always explain to an individual what you are doing, when you are assisting them.
29. Don't be in a hurry all the time. The more an individual can do for their self, the more dignity he/she feels.
30. Always remember everyone has feelings.
31. Always treat everyone as a separate person.
32. Assist an individual in areas where assistance is needed.
33. Do not yell, or scream at an individual. (Use a neutral tone)
34. Always dress an individual, per the weather.
35. Allow an individual to pick out his/her on clothes, if he/she can.
36. Do not talk about an individual to other people. (remember, confidentially)

37. Do not ignore an individual, when you know they are trying to get your attention.
38. Do not hit, or strike an individual at any time, or for any reason.
39. Do not invade an individual's space, (don't be all over them, when you don't need to be).
40. Make sure you always do your best for an individual.
41. Do not tell an individual you're going to do something and not do it.
42. Find out something about an individual before you start working with them.
43. Always look for a way to communicate with an individual even, if he/she cannot speak or have a hard time speaking.
44. Do not let an individual sit in a chair all day, and not check on him/her. (to see if he/she need to use the bathroom).
45. Do not let an individual sit around with dirty clothes on after a meal.
46. Make sure an individual can feed himself / herself before, you set a plate in front of them, and say eat.
47. Do not help yourself to things you see, lying around an individual room.
48. Do not leave an individual in their room unattended, when you are supposed to be taken care of them.
49. Do not allow an individual to lie in their rooms yelling, and screaming, because you feel they always do that.
50. Always knock on an individual door before entering.
51. Always identify yourself when entering an individual's room.
52. Always shut an individual door, when you are dressing them, and giving personal care.
53. Always avoid confrontation with an individual, because it can lead to behaviors.
54. Treat an individual like you would want to be treated, or like you want your family member to be treat.

55. Respect each individual right. They do have them even, if they living in a facility.
56. Be creative, when you are physical taking care of someone, people are different. (the same way may not work all the time).
57. Be flexible, change directions, or offer some other kind of assistance.
58. Be watchful of all your surroundings. (things can happen quickly)
59. Be very careful how you talk to an individual, (words can and do hurt).
60. Make sure you follow the procedure of the facility where you work.
61. When caring for a person that cannot get out of the bed, make sure you're doing what is require. (he/she may need to be turn every 2 hours to prevents bed sore, make sure you do that)
62. Do not be resentful, older people notice when you don't like your job.

Later, I went to work in a Psychiatric Hospital. The knowledge I gained in school made me aware of people with mental illness, emotional problems, and behaviors. School did not teach me all, I would need to know. School did not teach me techniques, and emergency codes, I would need to protect myself, and others from harm. While working in that hospital, I had to remember, I was working with people who had some type of mental problems, or emotional problem. Psychiatric work of a caregiver can be dangerous. The work can involve a lot of monitoring, searching, communicating, one on one care, and physical contact. They usually get discharge home or to a care facility. A lot of times, people are not what they appeal to be.

Let me give you one example; I was called a psychiatric technician. I was still taking care of people, just in a different way. I was making my rounds, and everything appealed to be quiet, all the patients appealed to be fine. The patients gathered around the table to get a cup of coffee. I was taking an account of who was drinking. I turned to walk away, and someone threw hot coffee in my face, thank goodness, the coffee wasn't hot. I later discover, the person who threw the coffee, was upset about something, that happened three days before. Whatever happen to the person, had nothing to do with me. I became the target of, the person anger. The person was physical restrained, and I had to remove myself from the situation. The patient was given medication.

I have seen medication do some wonderful things, working in mental health. I learned so much about diagnosis, mental illness, and that everyone has a breaking point. Pray you don't find yours. Psychology is one of those fields that makes you think and look at yourself. Under the right medication people can be as normal as you think you are. You should be disciplined when working with people with mental illness, because they can cause you to lose control. They could have, gone through some type of tragedy in their life, they could not deal with, death, drug problem, birth problems, and family problems, anything. All I'm saying, you can run across all kinds of reason people have mental problems, including their environment. Either way you look at it, they may need a caregiver, to watch over them, to make sure they don't hurt themselves, or others. Here are some do's and don'ts, I learned when I worked in mental health. You can combine this list, and some of the things from the preceding list to help you in this field also.

1. Things may not be what they appeal to be.
2. Always be alert to your surroundings know where everyone is.
3. Always be prepared to act, be ready for anything.
4. Never turn your back completely away from a patient.
5. Do not put yourself in a situation where you can't think.
6. Do not enter a patient's room without another staff knowing it.

7. Do not get yourself into a corner.
8. Never get angry with a patient, they may reverse it.
9. Never show fear or anxiety.
10. Never approach a patient in a defensive mood.
11. Always called assisted if you think there might be trouble.
12. Never take on more patience than you can handle.
13. Do not make yourself a victim.
14. When exiting, making sure a patient is not behind you, because someone can dart right pass you.
15. Work as a team. Keep all staff informed.
16. Make sure you are up to date on all techniques.
17. Always, document everything.
18. Be prepared to work very closely with a psychiatrist.
19. No, your limits.
20. All instructions should come from a doctor.
21. You must, always have control, and discipline.
22. Keep all information confidential, do not ask the patient personal information about themselves, let them freely tell you.
23. No fraternizing with the patients.
24. You may have to be a proactive person.
25. Do not get caught working by yourself.

The two lists helped me when I started working with another group of people. Individuals with Intellectual disabilities, a type of developmental disabilities. I worked with them in a community setting, or residential setting; they can range from having sever disabilities to mild disabilities. They needed assistance with their daily living skills, everyday life situation, from personal care, social care, physical care, health care, and community interactions. They might need assistance with their finance. Some of them needed assistance taking their medication. Caregivers who work with this population do a lot of prompting, redirecting, teaching, training, and some modeling. Some individual need to be taught, or showed how to express their feelings, or communicate things in a positive way. You may need to do some role playing with this group of individuals. When I say daily living skills, and assistance, here is a list of things I mean.

1. Personal hygiene (taking a bath/shower, brushing teeth, etc.)
2. Grooming (combing hair, dressing, etc.)
3. Cooking (knowing utensils, turning stove off, and on, preparing meals, using pots, and pans).
4. Cleaning (washing and putting away clothes, washing dishes, sweeping, mopping, vacuuming floor, etc.).
5. Shopping (buying food, clothes, house hold products, personal needs, etc.)
6. Paying bills (utility, rent, banking, personal bills).
7. Going to the doctor (getting good medical care).
8. Eating (assist with holding utensils).
9. Time management (getting everything done)
10. Safety (what to do in case of a fire).

Here is the list of do's, and don'ts, combine with the other lists, when working with individuals with Intellectual disabilities.

1. Use simple language when talking to individuals, (do not use fancy words you have learned in school, or from other professionals.
2. Look for change in behavior.
3. Have high expectations, (even if you found out the individual cannot do the job right now).
4. Focus on the individual you are working with not their disability, or the age of the person.
5. Monitor and document training.
6. Do safety training with the individuals.
7. Always use precaution when you are doing hands on care.

8. Be on the lookout for medical issues and report them.
9. Teach individuals about their rights.
10. Do not crowd them, let him/her come to you.
11. Do not force your ways, or beliefs on an individual.
12. Do not tell them what to do.
13. Do not intentionally aggravate an individual.
14. Make sure you always have the individual best interest.
15. You may have to make family contact.
16. Documents everything from giving aspirin to cough medication.
17. Report any marks, or bruise you see on an individual body, even if you cannot explain it.
18. Find out to whom you report abuse and neglect to.
19. Make sure you give everyone their right to dignity of risk.
20. Treat individuals like normal human beings. Don't make them feel different.
21. Get information about an individual, that would help you with their care.
22. If you are working with adults, treat them like adults.
23. The staff should not become part of a problem.
24. Do not take advantage of a situation.
25. Be accurate.
26. Be responsible for what you do.
27. Develop good communications skills.
28. Do not set the next staff up. Complete your assignment.
29. Do not set up a training program that is useless to the individual.
30. Do not use violence for control (pushing, pulling).
31. Do not show favoritism toward one individual over another.
32. Make sure an individual is appropriate dressed (weather-wise).
33. Be professional do not pick at an individual or make fun of them.

The biggest problem, I found when working with people with intellectual disability was the stereotyping. I cannot tell you, how many times; I have work with people, who think all adults people with intellectual disabilities act like children. Some people with intellectual disabilities are highly functional, and know exact what is going on. Some of them do not like it, so they start to act out in negative ways. Some of them can do, some things better than you, or I. As a caregiver, don't underestimate, or count this population of adults out. These three list may not apply to every adult you work with, because just like I said don't put people in a box. Everyone is different in their own way, but the lists can surely help you do your job better, no matter what population you're working with.

As you can see being a working caregiver is not an easy job. It is so much more involved than what you think, if you're going to be a good caregiver. So, if you have chosen caregiving as a career, don't listen to people when they say, all you do is that; I can do that with my eyes close. I am sure, if you are a caregiver, you have heard things like that more than once, I know I have. Believe me, if that was all you had to do, we would not need adult, and child protective serves, and there would be a lot of dead folks at the hands of their caregiver. If you have chosen to work as a caregiver, personally, or professional, be proud of it, if it's what you want to do. Don't forget you have chosen to take care of another human being.

THE LANGUAGE GAME

In this chapter, we will look at something else that can affect a working caregiver. It is what I call the "Language Game." This is the game where you should think before you write or document anything, because you could end up in a situation you don't want to be in. When you're working in a care facility, documentation is the last thing you think about; even though it is on the job description, (you must be able to write well and legible). Don't be surprised if your definition of writing well is different from the care facility definition of writing well. You think all you have to do, is write down what happened, or what you see. I have seen people lose their jobs, because of what they wrote. I called this a game because that's what it feels like when you go back, and forth with words. This game can also make you feel stupid. Sometime words change, and you don't know it, until you have to write/document something. Try to use words and phase that everyone can understand, if possible. Try to document things as soon as they happen, before you forget important information.

I went from saying, consumer, to clients, to residents, and now the correct word is individuals since 2010, it also can depend on the care facility. In some of these care facilities we used to say mentally retarded, and now the correct word is intellectual disabilities. Who knows what it will be in the next ten years? As I began to study, learn, and practice this game, I found my own way of understanding this language game. First, you would have to understand what I called the," you understood" words, and phrases. There are words, and phrases that are acceptable, and unacceptable in caregiving. Most unacceptable words, and phrases are the you understood words, and phrases. Those are words, and phrases you use when you're describing a situation, or telling what happened. Those are the words, and phrases that changes to acceptable words, or phrases.

For example, I pushed him out of the way. You cannot write "I pushed him." You may write something like, I assisted or escorted him out of the way. You understood "you pushed him", but you would not use the word "push" in your documentation, because it is a hard word, and it could indicate something negative, like force, anger, violence. Assisted or escorted is soft words that could mean help, guide, protect. All you're doing is using words, or phrases that describe a situation in a friendly, or safer way, not to cause conflicts. Don't think the people you work for, don't know this game. They just fail to tell you about it. This language game can be set up as the training tool to teach, and show people how to care for people, and document it. I found out the more I practice, and learn about this Language Game, the more I understand it. I learned more about what I could do, and write, or what I could not do, and write. Some people say "it is not what you say, but how you say it". The Language Game falls into that, it is not what you write, but how you write it. This kind of training can only be positive for a caregiver. Let's look more closely at this. Words, and phrases are continually changing in the caregiving field. This week, a word may be OK to write, but in three weeks, you may not be able to write it in your documentation anymore. There are many reasons words, or phrases are unacceptable in caregiving. One reason, certain words violate individual's rights. Another reason words can be threatening, and some of these words, and phrases imply violence, or punishment. Some words, or phrases could indicate abuse or neglect, be very careful with your language. Let's look at some possible examples in documentation for a working caregiver.

1. You have an individual who lives in a group home. Staff thinks this individual needs to go on a diet. Staff cooked fried chicken. The individual wanted a second piece. The individual got upset. Let's document this.
Today staff cooked fried chicken. Everyone was given one piece of chicken. One of the individual wanted a second piece. Staff told the individual he could not have any more. The individual got upset, and became verbally aggressive to staff. The staff told the individual to shut up, and that's when things get physical. Staff pushed the individual on the floor and forcefully held him there. While the individual was trying to move, he got a rug burn. This is what you wrote in your documentation.

First, your documentation is about a person, you would need the name. A lot of things in this incident was done wrong. You understood what you did. Most of the language that was use in this situation was unacceptable. How do you think this person can write this, to make it acceptable? Here is one way this incident could be written.

Staff fried chicken today, for dinner. Staff only fried enough for, everyone to get one piece. John wanted a second piece of chicken. Staff explained to John, there wasn't anymore. John got upset with staff, and became verbally and physically aggressive. Staff using an acceptable technique (named the technique in steps, what you did), lowered him to the floor. Staff stayed with him until he calmed down. While John was on the floor, he moved around, and got a rug burn. After, John calmed down, staff helped him get up off the floor, and tended to his injury.

Notice the language that describes this incident at the beginning. Then the language changed, when you had to make it an acceptable documentation. Look more closely at this documentation. You lower the individual to the floor, using a certain technique, (naming and describing the technique). The technique name could be, lowering to the floor. (describe technique in steps) Staff got behind the individual, put her arms around him, and lowered him to the floor. Staff stayed with him until he calmed down. This is not a real technique, but it is describing in steps. When documenting describes everything, if you say a person is upset, how do you know that? The person was crying, and screaming at everyone. That will give a picture of a person who is upset. Writing the wrong word can cost sometimes. If you use the words, he was verbally, and physically aggressive, what did he do? He was cursing, kicking, and throwing things at staff. I can picture he was verbally, and physically aggressive. Let's rewrite this documentation, and fill in everything, to see how it will read.

Staff fried chicken today, for dinner. Staff only fried enough for, everyone to get one piece. John wanted a second piece of chicken. Staff explained to John, there wasn't anymore. John got upset with staff, he started crying, and screaming at staff. He became verbally, and physically aggressive, John started cursing, kicking, and throwing things. Using the lowering to the floor technique; staff got behind John, and put her arms around him, lowered him to the floor. Staff stayed with him until he calmed down. While John was on the floor, he moved around, and got a rug burn. After John calmed down, staff helped him get up off the floor, and tended to his injury. This would be acceptable.

2. Mrs. No-Name was being very uncooperative with her caregiver. Her caregiver told her if she did not calm down she would not go shopping. That statement is unacceptable because, it violates Mrs. No-Name's rights. She is an adult, and she has the right to go shopping if she wants to. The caregiver decided she wasn't going to take Mrs. No-Name to the store, because she was acting up. You understood what happened, and what you said. Let's see if we can make some of these words acceptable for documentation.

   Mrs. No-Name, you need to calm down so you can go shopping. You basically said the same thing, but you used different words. You took out the phrase would not go, and replaced it with so you can go. In the first statement the caregiver was telling Mrs. N0-Name she was not going shopping. In the second statement, the caregiver was letting Mrs. No-Name decide whether she was going shopping. The essential point, Mrs. No-Name will not be going shopping if she does not calm down, don't forget, if you use words like uncooperative, acting out describe what the person is doing.

3. Mr. No-Name wanted to watch TV in the day. Staff told Mr. No-Name he had to watch what they were watching. Mr. No-Name got mad, and kicked the TV over. Staff grabbed him, and took him to his room, and locked the door. The way this is written now is unacceptable. Staff understood what she did. Let's make this an acceptable documentation.
   Mr. No-Name wanted to watch TV in the day room. Staff explained to Mr. No-Name, his other housemates were already watching a program; when they finished, he could pick a program to watch. Mr. No-Name did not like that, he became physically aggressive he kicked

the TV on the floor. Staff with open hands escorted Mr. No-Name to his room. He remained in his room, with the door open, under supervision. Staff continue to talk to him until he calmed down. See how the language changed. Staff grabbed him, and took him to his room, and locked the door; Changed to, Staff with open hands escorted Mr. No-Name to his room. He remained in his room, with the door open, under supervision.

4. Mr. So, you will be going to bed at 8:00 PM tonight, because you must get up early for your appointment. This statement was changed to; Mr. So, don't you want to go to bed at 8:00 p.m., so you can get up for your appointment in the morning?
The first statement sounded threatening, and the person told Mr. So, what he was going to do. In the second statement, Mr. So, will be making the decision.

5. Mrs. So, you had better get your shoes out of the middle of the floor, before I throw them away. This statement was changed to; Mrs. So, would you please get your shoes out of the middle of the floor, before someone trips over them?

The first statement was threatening. The second statement, Mrs. So, will make her decision. Always remember when you document use the words, and phrases that are nonthreatening, or violent. These are some words, and phrase, I think caregivers should avoid when documenting.

- Cursing words
- Threating words (you better, you will, I will show you, I make all the decisions around here, etc.)
- violent words (hitting, biting, pushing, pulling, killing, etc.).

- Aggressive words (hostility, offensive, and destructive), and (what I will do to you, etc.)
- Punishment, abusive, and neglectful words (no, you're not, go to your room, locked doors, why, and because). Why is the question, and because is the answer? Example, why can't I go to bed at 10:00 p.m. tonight? Because, you did not do what I told you to do.

Now let's look at some shift documentation. This is another part of the language game. You have incomplete documentation, and you have complete documentation. It is very important to do complete documentation, because it help the person, who comes on after you, and it can help if someone cannot speak. Completed documentation will cover you if something goes wrong during your shift. Complete documentation lets your supervisor know what is going on. Complete documentation can help a doctor found out what is going on with someone. You can catch medical, and behavior problem when you follow the documenting of a person.

Incomplete night shift; Individual was sleep when staff came in. Staff woke individual up to use the bathroom. Staff assisted individual with all his am care. Individual took his medication and ate his breakfast. Individual appeal to be in a good mood.

Completed night shift; J.D. was asleep when staff arrived, at 11:00 PM. At 2:00 am staff woke J.D. up to use the bathroom. He did not need any assistance in the bathroom. J.D. washed his hands, and went back to bed. 6:00 AM, J.D. was prompt to get up. J.D. was assisted with most of his am care (showering, dressing, combing hair, and brushing his teeth). J.D. was observed, by staff taking his am medication. J.D. was assisted with preparing breakfast, he ate pancakes this morning. After breakfast, J.D. cleaned his area (he put his plate in the dishwasher, and wiped the table down). J.D. appeal to be in a good mood, he was laughing, and talking to staff, and his roommate. J.D. said, he will be going out later this morning.

Incomplete 3-11 shift; Individual came home from her day program. She appealed to be in a bad mood. Individual ate dinner, and did all her pm care. She took her medication, and went to bed.

Completed 3 to 11 shift; Jan came home from her day program at 4:00 PM. She appealed to be in a bad mood, she was crying, and fussing. Staff asked her, what was wrong, and she said someone hit her. Staff talk to her, and calmed her down. She went to her room for a while. At 5:30 staff prompt her to get up, for dinner. After dinner, she refused to do her chores, because she had a headache. Jan completed her pm routine (shower, brushed her teeth). Jan got her sleeping clothes, and put them on. Staff assisted her with taking her pm medication. Jan was given a prn for her headache. Jan went to bed at 10:00pm.

incomplete 7-3 shift, individual did her own am care. the caregiver made her bed, and took her to breakfast. The individual ate a sandwich for lunch. The individual set in her TV room the rest of the afternoon.

Completed 7 to 3 shift, Sue got up this morning, and completed her a.m. care. Sue shower, and dressed herself. Staff assisted her with making her bed. Sue went out for breakfast at 9:00 A.M. with staff. Sue got back home at 10:30 AM. Sue went to the bathroom. Sue decided she wanted to set in the TV room until lunch, Sue read the newspaper while she was sating in the TV room. Staff assisted Sue with making a sandwich for lunch. After lunch, Sue was assisted, with going to her evening activity (bingo).

You can always write more. Try to use words, and phase that everyone can understand. Try to document important things as soon as they happen. Remember, make sure everything is clear, not confusing. Simple documentation can trip you up. You may say someone was crying today. You should explain why, and all the other details that surrounded the person crying. Some documentation can cause a lot of problems, if you are not clear.

This language game will encourage you to get some education, or training with documentation.

Most of the time; when you get a caregiver from an agency they do not have a lot of documentation to do. Most of the time an agency caregiver duties are straight to the point. If they come in to help you with personal care that's all they do. They might fill out some paperwork the agency requires. The person who hire the agency should sign off, saying the person did what he/she was supposed to do. Then you have those private duty caregivers. They do not come from an agency, most of the time a family member hires them. They do not have to document anything. The family just checked behind them to make sure he/she has done the job. In these situations, if documentation is necessary it is to make a complaint, or a praise about the caregiver.

The Formula for a Caregiver

Desir + Education + Training
= Experience = Sucess

While working as a caregiver, there were many times, I just wanted to quit, and do something else. Then, I saw something good come out of the work I did. Sometimes the good seemed little, and far between, but it felt good when it happened, and it kept me going. I was still determined to figure things out. I refused to believe money, and the work were the biggest reason people were quitting these types of jobs. I started thinking about the similarity, and the reason I found the job hard at first. I remember, when I worked with the elderly, some of them were very graceful, and some of them were not nice. Most of the elderly needed assistant with personal care, and physical care. A lot of them needed mobility assisted. Elderly care seemed to be straightforward, with few surprises. I found myself doing the same type of care in each care facility for the elderly. The difference was the people, and their personalities. The other different was the facility requirements, or expectation for you, and not having enough staff. Those are the things that made the job hard. When I worked with individuals with developmental disabilities, and intellectual disabilities, I had already learned about personal care. I was faced with things I knew nothing about, making doctors 'appointments, passing out medication, documentation, and following a lot of rules, and regulations. At that point everything I knew about developmental disabilities, and intellectual disabilities came out of books. I had no experience, or training. I had to learn to assist individuals in every aspect of their life, which include, preparing food, doing laundry, planning activities, and transporting. I had to pay close attention to each individual behavior, because he, or she may be trying to indicate something to you, like pain. I had to learn how to encourage, and build someone up. That is a hard thing to do, when you don't have the right attitude. Sometimes, if a person hears what they will be doing on the job, they may not take the job. Sometime a person take a caregiving job, and find out later, what they will be doing and quit, because, it can be overwhelming at first. I thought when I became a caregiver all I would have to do was take care of someone physical needs. I was wrong! See, I never got involved in the other types of care when I worked with the elderly in the nursing homes. The other types of care I am referring to are, social care, health care, and emotional care. I was providing social care and emotional care all the time, just did not know it.

Let me share my first interview, for a job working with developmental disabilities, and intellectual disabilities. First, the shift I applied for no longer existed, I did not find that out until the end of the interview. I was asked questions like; "did I have a problem lifting or feeding people?" They asked me, if I knew how to give a bath to someone, in a wheelchair. I could do those things. They told me one of the individual had behavior problems. I thought, how bad could that be? I knew something about behavior from school. They explained, I must do documentation. They also gave me a couple scenario. I had to explain how I would handle them, or what I would do to resolve the problem? They appeared to be common since scenario, also somethings I had learned in school. They wanted to know about my driving record, because I might have to transport someone. At the end of the interview, I was told the hours, and the shift I would be working. At that point it was nothing I could not live with. That interview did not last long, because I did not have any experience working with developmental disabilities, or intellectual disabilities. I did not know what questions to ask. Within three days I was offer the job, and I excepted.

Here are some things I learned after I started to work. I would be working by myself a lot. I had to learn basic first aid, CPR, and behavior management techniques. I had to take a medication test, and pass it, so I could administer medication to the individual living in the group home. I got nervous, and then more nervous; I learned one of the individual I would be working with had seizures. I never worked with anyone who had seizures. I was trying to figure out what they wanted from me. I knew nothing about seizures, or how to take care of someone with seizures. That job was taken my caregiver experience to another level. I thought about quitting, because I was afraid. I was told this individual could die from a seizure. The supervisor had another staff train me. This person did not know much about seizures either. The person told me all I had to do, was monitor, and document what happened. The person told me, move anything out of the way that he could hurt himself on while having a seizure. I thought that sounded stupid, because I wonder what he would be doing to make me move stuff. I constantly asked for some education, and training on seizures. The people in the facility knew they weren't hiring nurses or doctors. How would staff learned anything about seizures, if they did not offer some type of training? If you say someone might die from a seizure; I think it is irresponsible not to train, and education your staff. I wrote a letter, and complained a lot to other staff, and they agreed with me. After so much fuss was made, the people in the facility finally got some training and, education for staff. The people in the facility got a nurse to come in, and educate us, and do some training. The nurse was very good, after that training, I felt more comfortable working with individuals with seizures. They still did not inform new employees of the situation. Another individual had behavior problems. I don't mean those none violent behaviors, I learned about in school. This person, put his hands on you to hurt you. In- house training is importance, so you don't put people in danger. If I had known everything, I had to do, and deal with during the interview; I am not sure I would have accepted the job, with no experience or training. I lasted five years at that facility.

If these types of care facility gave in- house training and education in areas of important relating to the individual's living in their facility, they probably could save money, and time. For examples, if John Doe is schizophrenia wouldn't it be helpful to know something about schizophrenia, and his behaviors. If Jane Doe had a skin disorder, wouldn't it be helpful to know how to take care of her skin disorder. These are the types of care facility, where you, (the caregiver) make doctors' appointments, preparing food, do laundry, passing out medication, and do a lot of the documentation.

Care facility constantly spend money every time they hire a new group of people, especially when they hire people for the same position every three to twelve months. They may have to provide CPR, and first aid, and other training to each new employee, and if he/she doesn't stay, that is money lost for the company. The turnover rate in some of these types of care facility is unbelievable.

Even though, anybody can be a caregiver, should they? I think you need three things to make it as caregiver. I call these three things special qualities, and these special qualities are desire, education, and training, I think you would need these if you want to be a successful caregiver. Under these three qualities you may found other characteristics for example the quality, <u>desire</u> you may find words like (respect, compassion, honesty, love, like,). The quality, <u>education</u> you may find words like (knowledge, resource, understanding, skills). The quality, <u>training</u> you may find words like (experience, routine, practice, taught). Let's look at these special qualities one at a time, to see why I think they are so important. The first special quality is "Desire", it means to have a love, or strong liking for something, or someone, to have a strong feeling to do something, or be someone. I think this is the most important one, because it remind me of (Galatian 5: 22 to 23 fruit of the spirt) in the bible. I think a lot of good caregiver process the fruit of the spirt, or at least get close to it. This is the first thing a real caregiver should process, because if they don't they will not last. they should want to help people, not that they must, or it is their duty. I think some people have a gift for caring for other people. They are the first ones to offer you help, and follow through with it. If they are across a room, or a street, and they see someone struggling with something, they will consider going to the person aid. They may even go to the aid of someone they don't like. You need to have the desire first, and it will encourage you to move to the next quality, Desire along will not make you a successful caregiver working in a care facility. You will still need the other qualities. Let me give you an example, why just having the desire won't work by itself.

Some people think, because they have cared for loved ones, or friends they can care for anyone. This is untrue! I spoke to a lady who had just gotten a job working in a nursing home. She said, she took care of her mother for years. When her mother died, she decided to get a job working as a caregiver. She stated, she loves to care for people, and she was good at it. She felt being a caregiver was her calling. So, she started working in this nursing home as a caregiver. She explained, how she found herself in situation, she could not comprehend. She ran across families of people, she was taking care of; who were so rude, and she could not talk to them. She took care of individual who wanted to fight her, and were uncooperative. She knew nothing about rules, and regulations. She thought, all she had to know was, how to physically care, and personal care for someone. These were people she knew nothing about so, the care was different, and the way it was done was different. She found out she did not have what she needed to do this type of work outside of her home. She did things the way she knew how to do them. The people in the care facility didn't give her the training she needed to do the job their way, nor did they give her any information about the individuals she would be working with. On the job training, would have given her what she needed to do a decent job. She finally decided if the people in the care facility was not going to give her the training she needed, she would go back to school. She could, also find a caregiving job with a good training program. I think She had the desire, what she was lacking was education, and training. Let's look at education now.

"Education" is learning about your desire, and how to be put your desire to work. (I have the desire to be a cook, but I need to know what a cook is, and how to cook). I have the desire to play the piano. (I should learn everything about the piano, and how to play it). If your desire is to be a caregiver. (You should know who, and what a caregiver is). You should learn the rules, and regulation that are associated with being a caregiver. Learn about the people you might be working with, like the elderly, people with developmental disabilities, people with mental disorders. You will learn what developmental disabilities are, and what mental illness is. college will teach you theories, code of ethics. You will Learn how to communicate with people in different ways. College will give you the opportunity to practice as a caregiver. You may even learn some medical terms. You may even get a degree in a health care field (Human Services, Social Services, Psychology, Doctor, etc.). Some people think all you need is college to be a good caregiver, and be successful, but that is not to true.

I was working with a young girl; she had just gotten out of college. She took this job as a DSP until she could find another one. I think she major in psychology. She went through the whole song, and dance about how she wanted to work with people, with disabilities. She wanted to know what it was like to take care of them. She had not taken care of anyone yet. All she knew about caring for someone she learned in school, and what she saw other people do. She got her job, because of her educational background, she had no experience. She knew some guidelines, and she knew something about people. She knew about diagnosis, and behaviors. She knew a lot of stuff. What she learned later changed things. School taught her about behaviors, but it did not prepare her to deal with individual's behaviors, or what to do when she got in a situation. School taught her about diagnosis, but did not teach her how to work with people who had those diagnoses. School could not prepare her for the role she would be playing, when an individual was having an episode. School did not teach her how to protect herself, and others from harm. School is not going to tell you Mr. Doe has a problem with people looking at him, and if he catches you, he might hit you. School won't have that information about Mr. Doe. No book can tell you about the people you might be working with. The girl said, she did not go to college, to do this kind of work. I'm not sure this person had the desire. She lasted about three months. Most people who go to school, and get a degree in health care stay in the field of caregiving, but they look for something that doesn't involve a lot of hands on care, or situations. Most employers think if they hire someone with a degree they are getting the best, but in the caregiving field that is not always true. Your degree does not make you good at your job, it just let people know, you know the meaning of your job.

One time I got the flu, and ended up in the hospital; I was there a couple of days. I had a different nurse each shift; they check on you throughout the night. The night nurse took my temperature, I had a fever. The nurse said "O my god your temperature is 104 what to do". I watch the nurse pace for a minute, and put his hand on his head; it was a male nurse. I could not say anything, because I was feeling so bad, but I was thinking he was a nurse, what did he mean he did not know what to do. He called someone with more experience, and training. He may have the desire, he should have the education, but he did not have the last quality. In the real world, you just don't know what kind of situation, you might find yourself in. Education is wonderful, and we need it, having a degree is wonderful also, but sometimes you need more. These experiences prove to me education was not enough in the caregiving field. Let's look at the last special quality "training".

"Training" is practicing, developing, and perfecting, the things you have learned, putting your education, and desire to work. You may even learn new things during training. I learn how to cook, and went to work in a restaurant. I will be trained on how the restaurant is ran. (I will be able to practice, and perfect my cooking skills.) When it comes to caregiving, you train in several different areas. You begin to perfect your skills as a caregiver. There will be things, you need to know about everyone you take care of. For example, Mr. Doe, has a diagnosis of schizophrenia, you will need to know how it affects him. You will also get some training on how to work with people with schizophrenia. You will learn about the care facility rules, and regulations, proper procedures on protecting self, and others. You will be trained about your duties, and other things the care facility expect from you. This kind of information comes from on the job training.

Once, I had to train a new employee. I found myself saying things to her, I thought she would have already known from the interview. I asked her, how long she had been doing this type of work? She implied this was her first job as a caregiver. Then, I asked her about the work she did, before this job? She told me she was a waitress. I ask her if she had been a caregiver for anyone? She said "no". I ask her why she applied for this job? The lady stated she need a job paying more money, and taking care of someone can't be that hard. She then said she see people take care of people all the time. I must admit, that did not sound good to me, but I thought anybody could be trained to care for people. I tried to show, and explained things to her, about the care facility, and her duties. It is hard to train someone when he/she doesn't have an ideal about what he/she has gotten into. I don't think this person had the desire. She had a hard time understanding the documentation, and the language. She had a problem doing some of the work. She told me, she did not know taking care of people involve all this stuff. I explained to her, caregiving is different when you work in a care facility, from taking care of some in your home, or in their home. She said she probably will get her old job back, and go back to school. She did not like this kind of work. I don't think she had a problem dealing with people, she just did not have to deal with them on a personal level, and she felt this type of work was personal. If she had known something about caring for people, it would have helped her. She was lacking the desire, education, and the training in caregiving. She did not stick it out, she lasted over six months. She gained some education, and training during those months. You can see why just having one of the special quality is not enough, if you are going to make a successful career out of it. You might get by with two of the special quality, but can you imagine the experience, and success you would have if you process all three? Let's look at experience, and success.

Experience means you have spent time doing a job, in this case being a caregiver, and now you know what it takes to be a caregiver. You also process the knowledge about caregiving. Experience is something no one can take from you. Your experience can take you a long way, if you desire it. Sometimes your experience can lead you to a successful caregiving business, you can open your own care facility. You may even avoid some of the pit falls of opening a care facility. You can just take care of people in your own home, (a care provider). You can get a job in a care facility, and be a valuable employee to the company, and the individuals you serve. Sometimes you can run the job without supervision, because of your experience. If you want to, you can qualify for other position in the care facility. It is up to you, how much experience you want to have, and how far you want to go in the field. Remember, you don't have to go to college to get your education in caregiving, you just need a good training program that will give you some education as well. There are people who had the desire, and through a training programs they became good at being a caregiver. You can also work in different types of care facility without a lot of problems.

I think, without possession at least two of the three special qualities you are just a fair, or OK caregiver. When you are just a fair, or OK caregiver problems develop more quickly. You did not pay attention to any training, or you have no clue what being a caregiver means. I think the biggest problems that can develop is abuse, and neglect. I gave you the definition of abuse, and neglect in a previous chapter, but this is how it can look when you're working in a care facility. Sometime people abuse, or neglect someone, because they don't think it is abuse, or neglect, and they don't know any better, (lack of training). You can call someone out of their name, and this is mental abuse (stupid, crazy, dummy, old hagge etc.). You can hurt people by calling them names. (Words can hurt) If you send someone out in the cold, without a coat, or hat on, this is neglect. You failed to provide the proper clothes for the individual, some people don't think about things like that as a form of neglect. You failed to feed someone when you knew they could not feed them self. Then you have physical abuse, what people know more about. Like I said with education, and training you can cut down on abuse, and neglect. When working in a care facility, or being a care provider, you are constantly being watched for signs of abuse, and neglect. If you have any questions about abuse, or neglect ask someone, because education, and training on this subject is strongly recommended. The person who has the desire to do this type of work would seek understanding about abuse, and neglect. So, if you decide to go into the field of caregiving or become a care provider you should keep this formula in mind and I think you will have some success.

Let's look at this formula from a personal point of view. First, you should have the desire be a caregiver for a family member, friend, companion, or love one. Second, when you have the desire you seek education, because you want to know something about what you are dealing with. For example, if you are caring for someone with dementia, you want to know as much as you can about dementia. Once you educate yourself you start doing the work, and basically training yourself. That is how you get your experience as a caregiver on a personal level. You now have the desire, education, training, and experience. At this point, all you're missing is success. When you are a caregiver on a personal level, how do you measure success? Do you measure it by your education, and training, or do you base it on your desire, and experience? You can say you are successful because of your education, and training, some people would agree. You can think you are successful, because you have the desire to care for people, and you have been doing it for a while. The other thing about having success as a caregiver on a personal level, how well, or how serious you took what you were doing. You can get tired, and frustrated been a caregiver on a personal level, because of all the things you must do. Your desire can change to resentment, your education can be ignored, your training can be change to cutting corners, too, I don't want to do it. People can, and do mistreat their family member or love one when stuff like this starts to happen. They may not mean it, or sometime they may even justify it. Unbelievably, but some people mistreat their loved ones, because of something they may have done too them in the past. Some people may have other motives for mistreating their love one. Some people treat strangers better than they treat their love ones. So, be careful when you think your experience equal success in caregiving. The essential point is being true to the formula, sticking with it, and taken the necessary precautions to keep yourself from getting tired, and frustrated.

DESIER + EDUCATION + TRAINING = EXPERIENCE = SUCCESS

THE CARE OF INDIVIDUALS FROM A PROFESSIONAL LEVEL/ POINT OF VIEW

First, you get paid to be a caregiver on a professional level. You get a check for hours worked, from a care facility, a private agency, or an individual. This type of care comes with instructions, someone, or a group of people tells you what to do, and sometime how to do it. Each care facility has their own way of doing things. You must follow their instructions, and you may have some instructions from your state government you must follow also. Your first instruction is too complete the individual personal care (personal hygiene, grooming, dressing, etc.). The first thing you should do, if you do not know the person is look at his, or her chart, or ask questions about the person. You will be looking for personal information about the person you're taking care of. Information like the person name, how do the person communicate (talk, sign, gesture, etc.). Does the person walk, or is the person in a wheelchair? Can the person use his, or her arms, and hands? It will also tell you whether the person has mental problems, or other problems. This type of information lets you know whether the person can assist you. The things you should always want to do, if possible, encourage, and empower the person to do as much as he/

she can. Another reason for the information; the person may not want, or need your help with everything (dressing). The second part of your personal care is too report any changes, or problems with the person appearance (condition of the person skin, weight, eyes), and body functions (breathing, use of hand, arms, and legs). You also, need to look for changes in the person behavior (mental capacity, agitated, restless). You probably have some housekeeping duties as well (fixing the bed, and picking up things off the floor etc.). Something else you may have to do is prepared meals, or take the person to get their meal. You may have instruction on given medication, and transportation. You may have to transport an individual to and from a doctor's appointment. As a professional caregiver, you might have other duties as well.

Some care facilities provide other care like, social care. They have an activities department where residents can come together with their peers, and socialize, or play games. They provide health care, sometime a doctor come in to see the residents. Sometimes the facility provide transportation to and from the doctor office. They may have nurses, or LPN's to passing out medication. They provide mental care, and emotional care if needed. If a resident is going through some type of depression; the facility set up an appointment for the person to see a psychiatrist, or a social worker. Some care facilities have their own laundry department; people take the residents clothes wash and dry them.

In some other care facilities, the caregiver provides most of the social care. They come up with activities for the residents as a group, or individual. The caregiver provides emotional care by giving the resident one on one time. The caregiver encourages the residents to develop close community relationships, and family relationships. The caregiver may provide some of the health care. The caregiver pass out medication after they pass a medication management course. Most of the time they are the first person to notice medical problems. As a professional caregiver, the personal care rally changes from facility to facility. The way the care facility wants you or need you to do your job may be different. You still may provide some or all the physical care, social care, personal care, emotional care, health care, and other type of supports as needed. The last instruction you will follow as a professional caregiver is documentation. Each care facility has their own way of documenting. They might include some of the same information, but how you write it, or what you write may be different. You read in a previous chapter about documentation and how important it is. Also, remember if you are a caregiver for an agency you may or may not have to do a lot of documentation.

When working in someone home as a professional caregiver you followed the instructions of the person who hired you, or someone else in the home. Most of the time you don't have anyone telling you how to provide social care, personal care, physical care, emotional care, and health care. Most of the time you can decide how you are going to do the job he/she hired you to do. You still may do some cleaning, laundry, meal preparation, and transportation. You may have to make sure the person take his/her medication. When you work at someone's home the most important things for them, you are honest, respectful, reliable, and you are a safety conscious person. They also want to know; do you care about what you are doing? You will read about finding a caregiver in another chapter. The people you may take care of in a care facility, or a person home, are.

1. People with Alzheimer's, and dementia.
2. People with Developmental disabilities.
3. People with Intellectual disabilities.
4. People with Physical disabilities.
5. Elderly Person, who need assistant
6. People who have Family that is unable to take care of them or work.
7. People who are unable to take care of themselves.

8. People who are isolated, they don't have anyone to take care of them.
9. People with Chronic illness.
10. People with Mental Illness.

Whether you work in a big, or small care facility, or for one person do your best. If you don't possess any of the qualities of a caregiver at least care about the job. The people you take care of may have some health problems they may already have them, or they may develop them later. Here are some of the health problems you may encounter.

1. Seizures
2. Diabetes
3. Sleep apnea
4. Arthritis
5. Heart disease
6. Liver disease
7. Kidney disease
8. Allergies
9. Skin problem (Users)
10. Blind, and other problem associated with the eyes.
11. Ear, nose, and throat problems.
12. Destructive behaviors
13. Health problems that is associated with mental Illness
14. Alzheimer's and dementia.
15. Joints deterioration
16. Mobility

The Care of an Individuals from a Personal Level/ Point of View

When you care for someone on a personal level you do not receive a check, or pay for hours worked. Most of the time they are longer than normal hours. Another thing about personal level care, it is done in your home, or the home of the person you are taking care of. Caring for someone on a personal level takes your mind in many directions. You must make, and follow your own instructions. You must make your own schedule. You must prioritize things to make sure you get everything done that day. Your day probably starts with assisting, or providing physically, and personal care. This include giving bath/shower, dressing Grooming, and dental care. The next thing you do, is fix the person's meal (breakfast, lunch, dinner). You are that person companion, friend, loved one or concern family member. When it comes to the personal level/point of view of care, you probably go beyond the professional level, because you are doing it all. You don't have the help, or assistant you may get when working in a care facility. You're basic on your own, if you cannot call someone to help you. This is just the start; you are responsible for seeing that the person heath needs are met. This could include making medical appointments. Deciding on what medical appointments need to be made, and follow up on appointments. You make sure the person has his/her medication. and you make sure the person takes their medication. You are responsible for the safety of the person; you make sure the person is in a safe environment. You may have to do some pulling, and lifting by yourself. If you are caring for someone who cannot get out of the bed you may have to turn that person several times a day to prevent skin breakdown. You are the housekeeper also. These things can be hard work, and they can take a tool on your body.

Another thing about being a caregiver from a personal level/point of view is your mind. When it comes to your mind, you must decide whether you are, or if you want to become the person caregiver. You must decide, if you have the time, and the space. You should think about the kind of caregiver you will be. You should think about the changes, you might have to make in your life, and how those changes will affect you. You must take your health in consideration. You must think about your other family members, and how your decision to become the person caregiver will affect them. In your mind, you might think you should do it, because there is no one else.

Your feeling is another thing that can get to you when it comes to the personal level of care. You may feel it is your responsibility, or obligation to take care of the person. When you feel that way it is usually a loved one (parent, child, spouse, or companion). Most likely those are the people other family member expect you to take care of. You may feel you're not doing a good job no matter how hard you try. After a while you may feel being a caregiver is not for you, and you don't want to do it anymore. You are so tired you're afraid you will do something wrong. You start to feel all kinds of emotions, (crying, angry, frustrated, sad, confused, fearful, worried, scared, depressed, hopeless, sorrow, and uncertain).

Guilt is the biggest, and worst feeling, you start to experience. You feel guilty, because you don't want to take care of the person anymore. You feel guilty, because you have to work. You feel guilty, because you don't have the space. You feel guilty, because you do not have any help. You feel guilty, because you're making all the wrong decisions. You feel guilty, because you're coming up with reasons, or excuses why you can't be the person caregiver. Other family members make you feel guilty. You're forced to put your loved one in a care facility, and you feel guilty about that. Guilt makes you visit your loved one constantly, and fuss about everything that is going on in the care facility. Nothing staff does will satisfy you. You expect everything to be perfect, because you're feeling guilty. Staff must put up with your feelings, and emotions. Not to say some of your concerns are not real, but it may be the way you present them. When you are fighting on behalf of your loved one, family, or friend, it is not to ease your guilt or pain, but to make life better for him/her.

The same people you take care of on a personal level are the same people you take care of on a professional level. You can see the list on page 76 and 77. They may have the same health problems, see list on page 77. Two important differences between a professional caregiver, and personal caregiver. One, a professional caregiver gets to go home after their shift is over. Nine times out of ten the personal caregiver is already at home, and it is hard to get a break. Two, safety, free from any type of abuse, or neglect. The professional caregiver has many people watching out for abuse, and neglect. Most of the time the personal caregivers do not have anybody watching out for abuse, and neglect, unfortunate it does happen on the personal level more often then we care to know. You may not believe it, but being a caregiver on a personal level abuse, and neglect can go on for years, and never get reported.

Looking for a Care Facility

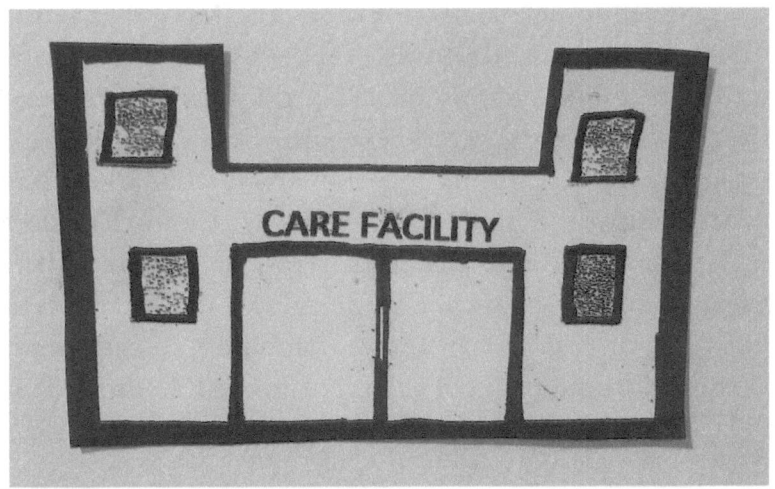

No matter what, and how people feel about care facilities, we need them. Remember, some reasons we need care facilities, some people do not have anyone to take care of them, when they need it. Some people don't want the responsibility of taking care of anyone. Some people are not in a place to take care of anyone. Some people are unable to take care of anyone. Some people don't have the time to take care of anybody. Some people cannot afford to take care of anyone. I am sure there are many other reasons.

There is all size of care facilities. You got those big care facilities that have 50 plus individual living in them. Those facilities are license by the government, and mostly ran by the government. Then, you got those small privately ran care facilities that may have 4-15 individuals living in them. These facilities also should be license by the government. When the government licenses you, all those rules, and regulations must be follow, by the facility, and its employees. First let's look at some different types of care facilities you might want to consider. They may have different names, but they all provide care, and service to people in need. Some of the care, and service may be specialized for a certain population of people, (the elderly, children, developmental disabilities, intellectual disabilities, mental health, or mental Illness). I looked up some of different types of care facilities. Some of the definitions ran so close together, I was not sure what type of facility I was looking at. So, I pieced the definitions together from what I knew about the care facility, and my experience with them. I noticed in some circumstances the different types of care facilities are interchangeable for example, some people call a group home (adult home, or residential home) some people call a nursing home (group home or a convalescent home). Let's see if I can simplify it just a little.

1. Assistant living- Housing for the elderly or person with disabilities who may need help in certain areas of their daily living. They do not need nursing home care. They are mostly mentally function, but may have physical challenges. They may be part of a retirement community, senior citizen housing complex, or they may stand alone. They continue to do their own things, and they are license.

2. Group Home /Adult Home - can be a private resident for children, or adults who cannot live on their own, or

do not have anyone to care for them. There are no more than 4 to 6 individuals living in the home. they have professional caregivers taking care of them 24 hours a day. They get assistance with all their daily needs. They may have mental challenges. They have a lot of in house activities. They are license

3. Nursing Home/Convalescent Home -A private, or public long-term care facility for the elderly who is unable to care for themselves. They might be suffering from chronic illness, major physical challenges, or disabilities. They cannot live with family. They may have in house activities, and they are license.

4. Residential Homes/ Group Home- A long-term private ran home, or a state ran home. They are in regular neighborhoods. They have 4 to 6 individuals living in the home. They serve adults, and children with developmental disabilities, and intellectual disabilities. they have personalized service, and care, which is called person center. Most of their caregivers are called Direct Support Professionals (DSP). They provide service in every area of the individual's life, by training, educating, and assisting the individual to live as independent as possible. They have in house, and community activities. They operate 24 hours a day, and they are license.

5. Adult Day Care/Adult Day Program/Adult Center- A place where people with developmental disabilities, intellectual disabilities, other disabilities, and the elderly can attend during the day. Under the care of a licensed professional who are fully capable of taking care of them. The place is staff with other qualified workers to assist. These centers give the individuals a chance to get out into the community, and socialize. A place that gives

the individuals a sense of worth by providing activities. These centers give caregivers a break. They are license. For more information about these care facilities contact the facility directly.

It is hard for some people to put a love one, or a family member in a nursing home, or any other type of care facility. It's even harder when you don't have the money, or the time to look for one. You can't afford those luxurious places you see on TV. You can't even afford a real good one. So, you get discouraged, and look for ones that range from nice to fair. When you find a care facility, you don't ask too many questions, or you don't know what questions to ask. You make a choice, or decision based on your finance, or the person finance, this may not be the best thing to do. You may find out later that the money you saved wasn't worth it. Your love one, or family member has gotten hurt. Every time you visit your love one, or family member he/she was lying in a wet bed, or unclean. You found out, the place doesn't have enough staff to take care of your loved one, or family member needs. The money you think you saved might be needed for emergency care, or placement until you find another place. It is better to find a suitable place at the beginning, and not base your decision solely on finance. How much a place coast is something to keep in mind, but you also want a place that is going to take care of your love one, or family member. You also, want a place that is going to keep them safe. Let me share two situations where the family found out they had chosen the wrong place.

I did some volunteer work at a group home when I was in college. It wasn't a very good place; the truth it turned out to be a very poor place. They needed a lot of help, and I wanted to help. This place passed out cigarettes to the individuals living there every hour. Someone would yell "cigarette time" they all came running. I thought everyone smoke! One day a woman was visiting her mother. We all were sitting outside; it was a warm day. The woman, and her mother did not appear to be talking to each other, they were just sitting there. A staff came out, and yelled "cigarette time" the women's mother got up, and got in line to get her cigarette. I looked at the daughter, and she was shaking her head as if she did not like it. I walked over to the daughter, and started talking to her. She told me her mother never smoked a cigarette in her life, until she came to this place. I did not say anything, but it started me thinking. I decided to watch some of the individual during smoking time. I saw a lot of people put the cigarette in their mouth, and just puff, and blow spontaneously. After a few puffs, and blows they threw the cigarette a way. So, I figure most of these people did not smoke. The next time they called cigarette time, I was standing there, everyone ran, and got in line for their cigarette. When they got to people I saw puff, and blow I said, "you don't smoke"? Some of them got mad, and some of them got out of the line, the woman's mother got out of the line. It was clear they did not smoke, but when I walked away some of them got back in the line including the woman's mother. I said to the staff; "a lot of these people, don't smoke". The staff said "I know". I asked "why do you give them cigarettes"? The staff implied it gives them something to do, and they look forward to it. That confused me. I felt the place was promoting bad habits, and health problems, and they did not seem to care. I tried to talk to the administrator about it. She just did not care about my concerns. I was just a volunteer. I spoke to the daughter again, and she told me she was looking for another place for her mother. She also talked about the extra money she had to spend. She got to buy, her mother a whole new wardrobe, because the facility doesn't know what happens to her clothes. Three years later I found out the state closed that facility down. Like I said, it wasn't a nice place, but it was inexpensive. The money the daughter saved cost her at the end. She had to find a temporary placement for her mother, until she finds a suitable place. Let's look at another example, of how you can choose the wrong place.

I spoke to a woman, who put her father in a nursing home, I wanted to know how she went about it. She said, she found some names in the telephone book, and just called them. She did not know what she was looking for in a nursing home. She said, she needed a place that could take care of her father. She chose the cheapest home she could find. She went, and talked to the administrator, then she filled out an application. She did not look the place over, or ask any important questions. She made a very big mistake. Her father was in good health, but he could not walk, and he needed assistance with his personal care. Someone in his family would visit him every other weekend. For the first couple of months, her father appealed to be doing fine, suddenly, he started to lose weight. The family notice he was looking smaller every time they visit. A family member asked why was he losing weight. Staff said, he was losing weight, because he was not eating a lot, and he also had a cold that lasted a while. The family was OK with that. A couple of weeks later, the woman got a call from the nursing home, saying they had to take her father to the hospital. The doctors said he had the flu, and they found sores on his back side. The woman got mad, and started cursing at the administrator. She wanted to know how this could have happened. She wanted to bring a suit against the facility, but she decided not to. She just wanted to get her father out of there, and find another place. She found another place, but she still did not know what she was looking for. I ask her if she thought a guideline on how to choose a care facility would have helped her. She said "yes", and she probably would have made better choices, when looking for a care facility. Her father passed away within two years after he got in the second facility.

Know, I want to share my personal experience, about not making the right decision when it comes to choosing a care facility for my mother. Like I mention earlier when you're personal involved your feelings, emotions, and everything get twisted up in your mind. Sometimes things happen so fast you cannot think. My mother had been in the hospital two weeks, and three days before she was going to be discharge; the doctor talked to us, and said she would needs some rehabilitation. He recommended my mother go to a rehabilitation center, just long enough to get back on her feet. My mother still could make her own decision at this point, but she would always say, what every you think. My mother knew I was going to take good care of her. So, the family left all the decisions up to me, when it came to our mother's care. I was not happy with what the doctor said, but I thought if it was going to make my mother better, I would go along with it. Things were happening so fast I did not have time to check around for rehabilitation centers, so, I let the hospital chose one for me. I thought if the people in the hospital recommended the facility it had to be a good one. I did not ask any questions, that was wrong. I knew better from my experience working in some of those care facilities, but I could not think, it was my mother. The rehabilitation center was connected to a nursing home. My mother would stay in the nursing home, and receive rehabilitation service during the day. The hospital staff handle the transfer, and the transportation. My mother was all settle in her room by 3:00 pm that evening. They gave her something to eat, and ask us some questions. About 8:00 pm my mother needed to be changed, she had use the bathroom on herself, at this point she was not walking. I called a staff, she told me after she finish, what she was doing she would be right there. I understood so, my mother, and I waited patiently. My mother room had started smelling, so about 8:30 pm I called the staff a second time. I had to call the staff a third time. Staff finally get in the room at 9:00 pm. She asked, what did we need? I explained to her my mother need to be changed. She told me she had to get some things, and she would be right back. I had to leave, and I trusted the staff to do what she said she was going to do. I told my mother to call again if the staff did not come. While I was at home getting dressed for work, I felt very uneasy about the facility. I knew I should have asked questions.

I was on my way to work, and something just told me, go to the nursing home. I showed up at 11:00 pm that night. I did not see anyone at the front desk, so I went straight to my mother's room. My mother was still lying in urine, and feces. I asked my mother did someone change you, she shook her head no, my mother did not look well at all. The room was smelling terrible. My mother was howling in pain. I had to walk up, and down the hall to find someone. The staff told me my mother had been changed. We went to my mother's room, I showed her the stains on the sheets where it had been dried up, and wet repeatedly. She told me she was going to report the staff. I stayed there until my mother was clean. I kept my cool, because I felt I was partly at fault. I did not check the place out. I did not do what I knew how to do. When I talked to the administrator she seems to take it lightly, and made excuses for staff, at that point I acted like a fool, I lost it. I removed my mother from that care facility the next day. I decided her rehabilitation would take place at home. I contacted the necessary people, they came to my home, and work with her. If I had done my homework in the first place, I wouldn't have gone through that situation with the facility. I wasted money, and time. I had to pay for transportation to the care facility, and one night stay. The time that was spent letting the hospital find a care facility, I could have been doing my homework. The facility did not have enough staff to do the work. Staff was not held accountable. Some of the staff did not take their job serious. There was other negative thing about the facility. When you don't have a clue about care facility, and you don't take the time to check them out, those are just a few things that can happen. Like I mention, one of the biggest problem in finding a care facility is money. Even expensive care facilities have problems so, don't think just because you pay a lot of money to a care facility you get better treatment. Remember people work at these care facilities, and some time they move from facility to facility. It does not matter what type of care facility you choose everyone deserves good care, and you need to expected it. Don't forget a lot of bad care comes from the lack of the three qualities desire, education, and training. There are things you should do, and question you asks before considering a care facility, no matter the cost.

1. Conduct your own background check, start with the Better Business Bureau?
2. Consider the location.
3. Check the facility license.
4. Check for allegations of abuse.
5. Ask about staffing.
6. Visit the facility at least three times before you decide. Do not visit at the same time?
7. Look at the facility mission and vision statement.
8. Ask the administrator how they ensure staffs follow the mission and vision statement?
9. Talk to other people who has a family member living in the facility.
10. Look at the appearance of the facility and the individuals who live there.
11. Do they have a housekeeping department?
12. Observe the interaction with the resident and the staff.
13. Ask about their dietary department, if they do not have one, you want to know how the resident gets their meals.
14. How are doctors' appointments handle?
15. How are personal items handle? Who purchase them?
16. Do they have an activity department, or do they have any activities doing the week? This is very important. It may not seem like it, but look at the cigarette incident I spoke about earlier. Everybody enjoy activity. Even if it is just something to look forward to. Activities also help with depression so, a doctor said.
17. Make sure the facility can meet your family needs.
18. Does the administrator keep check on what is going on in the facility?

19. How often are the residents check doing the night?
20. Ask any other question that come to your mind no matter how it may sound.

once you have decided on a care facility there are still things you should do and questions you should ask. This is an ongoing thing.

1. Give as much information as you can about the person, who will be living in the facility. Sometimes the more staff knows about a person the better care they can receive.
2. Make sure your family clothes are kept clean, and kept up with.
3. Visit your family member different times of the day and different days of the week.
4. Let the facility know you will be involved in your family member care.
5. Notice the difference from announced visits to unannounced visits.
6. Make sure one of your visits is at meal time. If the facility has a cafeteria you should eat with them, it will let you know how the food taste, and what your family member is eating.
7. How often does staff check on the residents?
8. When visiting check your family member bed room for cleanness.
9. Check your family member for signs of abuse or neglect (remember the definition).
10. At least once a month or sooner inventory family member belonging.
11. Monitor your family member care.
12. Continued to question things that looks out of place.
13. Every so often, you should meet with the administrator (4 to 5 months), to talk about your family member.

These things do not guarantee you're going to find the perfect place, but it will give you an ideal of what to look for, and what not to look for. This is a hard decision for a lot of people, so don't take it lightly. Take your time, start doing your research as soon as it looks like you might be moving toward that direction. Try not to look for a care facility when you are stressed out, or burned out, because it makes you take the first place you see. Try not to look for a care facility when you are feeling guilty, because that makes you look for places you cannot afford. Guilt makes you hard to please, because no matter what place you choose good, or bad nothing they do will be right. You become a dissatisfied family member instead of a concern family member.

It is important that you choose the right care facility, for your family member. Other tips, if the person you are considering placing in a care facility is of sound mind, and can make decision, ask him/her to help you. It will make your family member, and you feel better. It also will let you know how the person really feels about living in a care facility. It will help you get rid of, some guilty feeling. You can contact an agency, that will help you find a care facility. The agency will do most of the stuff for you, like background check, to see what other people have said about the facility. They will check if the facility is license. Remember, you still need to do your part, because the agency will not be at the interview, and they will not watch over your family member. Also, when you are looking for a care facility other family members may have an opinion. You may run across family members, that do not agree with you putting the person in a care facility. Most of the time those are the family members who say, they will help, but never do, or they disappear when you need them. If you are responsible for making decisions, and taking care of your family member, you should do what is best for you, and your family member. Do not beat yourself up, because you feel the best, and safest place for your family member is a care facility. I cannot say it enough, just do it right.

LOOKING FOR A CAREGIVER OR NEEDING A CAREGIVER

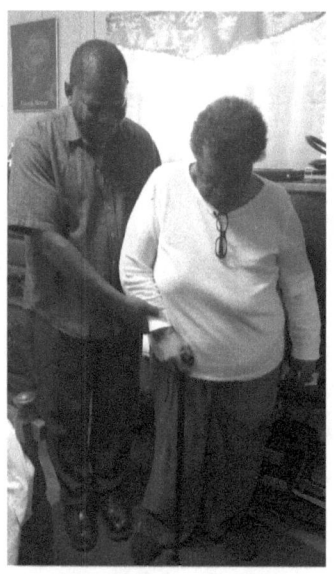

We all know, no one is perfect, and it is hard to find the perfect job, but as an employee in a company we should do our best. Some companies do not pay a lot of attention to mistakes, because they can be fixed. Some companies can go back to the drawing board, and change the planes. Some jobs, don't require you, to have a good personality, patients, understanding, caring heart, or even be creativity. Some jobs do not require you to work with people, and the public. There is a job, where you need to have these things, and a lot more, and you also, work with people, and the public. It's a job where mistakes can hurt, and have serious consequences. This is a job where your judgment or lack of judgment can come back to haunt you. This job is called caregiving, and you are the caregiver. Sometimes people need a caregiver to work in their home. You decide you do not want to put your loved one, or family member in a care facility, but you will need help from a caregiver. The person looking for a caregiver, should have the same frame of mind as the person looking for a care facility. You need to do some work. Do not give up your control. Do not let your feelings, and emotions run you (be assertive). Do not pick a friend, or family member to be your caregiver for pay, it just gets messy.

Sometimes your insurance will provide a caregiver for you, it might be a part of your insurance package. This makes things easy for you, you don't have to worry about finance, you should check the person out for yourself. Keep your control. If you don't have anyone providing a caregiver for you, go through an agency, if possible. The agency will provide a caregiver for you. The company might have another name for their caregivers, but you know what they do.

An agency should have already done the hard part for you, like background check, work experience, and reference check; make sure the agency has done those things. If the agency has not done those things, when they percent you with a person, you do not want to deal with them. Always ask the agency questions about, the person they are sending you, that is another way of finding out whether the agency has done their job. An important question to ask is, how long the person has worked for your agency. This is the reason I think that question, is important. When you have a new employee (from one to four years), he/she will do the best work, or he/ she will leave the company within that period. Another reason, a new employee does good work, is he/she wants to look good, or he/she wants to advance quickly. They tend to do their best, and go beyond their job description. Then you have the older employees, the ones who have been working for ten years or more. They will do a good job for you, because they have gotten use to the work, and what they are supposed to do. They have come up with good ideals, on how to do the job easier, or better. They have gained a lot of knowledge, about what they do. Those are the employees that might retire from the company. The next group of employees are those, I call middle employees. They are the ones who have been working for the company five to nine years, and some of them do a fair to poor work. The middle employees are not sure how much longer he/she can do this type of work. They are not sure how much longer he/she will be there, and he/she is probably looking for another job. They might decide caregiving is not for them, or they don't like the agency. They will not leave the job, until they have find another one, so they unhappily stay there. Whatever reason, you have the most problems out of these employees. Also, knowing how long an employee has been with a company gives you a glance at how serious they are, and their work experience. Let the agency know your concerns.

Sometimes people cannot afford to go through an agency, so they find a caregiver on their own. So, if you do not go through an agency make a list of things you need to do, and question you need to ask. You will need to do this if you are going to find a suitable caregiver. Your list could look something like this:

- Get a simple application that ask the basic questions, and add the question, you may ask a caregiver. You can also, make up an application that fits your need (see an example on page 102 - 105).
- Spend the money on a background check, but be aware that a background check doesn't give you all the information you would need to hire the person. (Be safe)

- Verified the person's identity, make sure you see a picture ID.
- Be very clear, and direct about what you want, and the type of person you want to be in your home.
- Don't be impressed by a nice smile, or the phrase, "I like helping people".
- Accept work experience, reference, and personal letter reference. Personal letter reference is used, when your only experience is personal. You should have two letters, and the letters should come from people who know you did the work. (make sure you check all reference).
- Have an ideal, how much caregiving experience you want the person to have. If they do not have any, move along.
- If your family member is still able to go out, make sure you hire a person who doesn't mind going out, or driving.
- If something doesn't look, or sound right check it out, or watch everything.

Make sure you look at the application closely, and make sure the dates on the application, and reference matches. Let's look at the power of the application more closely. You know an application will not guarantee you anything, especially if the person has lied, and has gotten others to lie. You can do everything right, but something can still fall through the cracks. You can think you have the right person on paper. Never the less, the application gives you power; if you need to take the person to court, and you have done your job. You will have all the information needed to prove you case. An application might make it easier to track the person down. An application makes the person accountable for the information. Your application does not have to look like the one in this book. It is your decision, whether you even need, or want an application. I think it is important to get some information about the person you will bring into your home.

Remember, I said do not hire family members, or friends. The key word is hire. You trust them, so you'll going to give them more freedom to your house. You're probably less open with them, about what you want. Whatever you think can go wrong, will go wrong. You do not want to take your family member, or friend to court. It will involve other people, and it can divide, or break up families, and friendship. If possible stay away from that situation. Now, if they want to volunteer to help you, that's something else.

When you have decided on a caregiver, listen to the person who needs the care, if he/she can understand. Usually, the person who hire the caregiver wants help at the cheapest price. So, most of the time, they do what they want to do, and do not consider the person needing the care. They seldom pay close attention to the quality of care, that is going on, but the person who is receiving the care of does. Everything the person says about the caregiver may, or may not be true, but it is your responsibility to check. Never discourage the person receiving the care from voicing their opinion about something they feel is wrong. You can discourage a person by saying things like you don't like anyone; you don't like the sex, or the color of the person skin; you complain about everything; if you don't stop complaining, I will leave you here along; if you are not quiet, I just might put you in a home; I don't believe anything you say. Talk like that makes a person clam up, and become afraid to say anything, and what you don't know can hurt. That is how abuse, and neglect happens on a personal level. Do not give the caregiver total control, because bad things can be happening right in your home. Be actively involved in the type of care that is going on. Ask questions if you do not know what the caregiver is doing. Complain if things are not going right. Don't worry about your complaining, because if you show you are interested in what is going on, the caregiver will watch what he/she does. You should never fear retaliation, because if a caregiver retaliates, it only makes the problem worse, and it could end up in court.

Remember, no matter how much money you pay for caregiving service, the care is supposed to be the same. Each person should be treated with dignity, and respect. Each person should be free from abuse, and neglect.

I this section, I would like to stress why being actively involved in the care of your family member, or friend is so important. Make the caregiver feel like a camera is in every room. It has been said more than once, people tend to be more careful when they think someone is watching them. There are people who do not have anyone watching over them. You can be a represented/advocate for someone receiving care, who do not have anyone watching over them. You can perform these duties in a care facility, your home, or another person home. A facility can also be actively involved in the care of their clients. Don't just say you are, be real about it. You would be surprised at the things you could stop from happening, when you are actively involved. The best way I can explain this is to tell you a couple of stories. First, let's define what actively involve, represented and advocate means.

Actively involved, is when you are closely involved in something, in this case a person's life. You participate in their wellbeing, you may have to visit them often. You must keep a watch on everything (vigilant). You may be that person eyes, ears, and voice.

Represented, A person who represent someone. A person who speak, or act on another person behalf, (client). Lawyer, friend, another caregiver. The person that must be notified if something is wrong with the client, or if something happens to the client.

Advocate, the person who will argues for the clients (better treatment, better living arrangement, better care etc.).

John work as a caregiver in a nursing home; he had been an employee five years. John consider himself a good employee, and he had a good work record. The facility could always count on him. He would fill in when they were short staff, and he never complained. John proved he could do good work. His clients were always taking care of. The nursing home has thirty employees working as caregivers. Out of the thirty employees, there were six males, and they were very valuable. They could help with lifting, and with the male clients. John had about three years of experience prior to getting the job at the nursing home. John had a total of seven years' experience working in this field at the time of this incident. The facility operated twenty-four hours a day. They served one hundred clients. Fourteen employees work on the morning shift, ten was on the evening shift, and six was on the overnight shift. Only the caregivers worked the overnight shift. John regular shift was the evening shift (3:00 PM to 11:00 PM). One day, John was asked to stay over, and work the overnight shift (11:00 PM to 7:00 AM). They had two people to call out. The home could not risk being short two staff, so John took the shift. John finished his first shift, and went straight into his night shift. The night was quiet. All the clients were in bed. Staff had to do their regular bathroom checks. About 3:00 AM., staff started taking their breaks. John took his break about 4:00 A.M. Around 4:40 AM staff noticed John had not come back from break. One staff said, "he's properly somewhere sleeping, because he was doing a double". Another staff said, "let him sleep, we will find him when it is time to do the last check, if he is not back.

It was 6:00 AM, and John Still had not showed up. Two staff started looking for him. They checked the staff lounge, looked outside, and in his car. John was nowhere to be found. One staff said "he must have fallen asleep in one of the client's room. First, they called him on the loudspeaker, but they did not want to wake any of the clients up. They decided to go room to room. At 6:15 AM, John was found lying in a client's bed sleep, the client was a female. The staff just stood there in shock, not know what to do, she called another staff, and they both stood there in shock. They though he was going to wake up, but he did not. They noticed his pants were loose. The staff decided to go back to the front, and call him over the loudspeaker again. They both were afraid, and nervous, because they knew what they had to do. John responded to the loudspeaker that time. He came to the front like nothing was wrong. Another staff asked him where he was? John stated he was sleep on the back patio. The two staff did not even look at him. They knew they had to report him. One of the staff went into an office, and call the supervisor. The supervisor told staffs not to say word. She needed them to stay there until she got there. It was 7:00 AM, and the shift was over. John said good-bye. The two ladies acted like they had work, they needed to finish. The supervisor got there at 7:30 AM; she asked the two staff to come back to her office. She took their statement, and informed them not to say a word to anyone, if they did their job could be on the line as well. The supervisor told the ladies they could go home, and she could take it from here.

John had not been seen in a couple of days. The two ladies knew, John was let go, but they did not know what happens. John had a lot of friends on the job so, the ladies was sure he had contacted them. The rumors that was circulating said, John was given the opportunity to resign, because he was sleep on the night shift. The two ladies were upset, because they let John resign, and keep his reputation intact. Everything was handle in house, and John work experiences still looks good. John walked away able to get another job in another facility as a caregiver (this is bad). That facility put other people at risk. This kind of practice happen more often than people know; facility don't want to mess up their reputation. They allow people who are not suitable to be a caregiver a chance to walk away; when it appeared, they may have committed abuse, or neglect.

Who knows how long John has been doing something like this, and what else has he done? One reason John got away with this, the lady(client) did not have any family, or a represented/advocate actively involved in her life, and care. An actively involved person would look for any changes, physically, or mentally. They might even notice the condition of a person room. An active person would be so involved in the client care, a caregiver would think hard before he, or she does anything wrong. An actively involved person may have requested criminal charges, brought against John. John got away with it, but people like John don't stop. The law must stop them. Remember, a John could be working in your facility or even in your home.

I was talking to a woman in her forties, she was the caregiver for a family member (her Aunt) which was her father's sister. The aunt had no other family. She said, she tried to care for her aunt by herself. She had no real experience, just a caring heart, and she felt she was supposed to do it. The woman was still trying to work a full-time job. Things start to get very hard for her, and she was physically wearing down. She started asking people if they knew anybody who did caregiving work. Someone told her about a person, who did private duty work for people. The woman got the person name, and number, she called, and they set up a meeting. They talked about 30 minutes, the woman told the caregiver, what she was looking for. She told the caregiver her aunt needed assistance with everything. She would have to fix breakfast, and lunch. She would have to do some housekeeping, and laundry. The woman also told the caregiver, her aunt could communicate, and she had no problem letting anyone know what she wanted, or what she did not want. The women asked the person about her experience as a caregiver, how much she charged, and the hours she could work. The woman felt the person was nice, she smiled a lot, and said, she just loved doing this type of work. The caregiver, said she love to work with people who could tell you, what they want, and you don't have to guess. The woman fell for it, they agreed on a price, and the date the person was to start. The person worked for the woman about two months, and everything appeal to be going very well. The aunt, and the caregiver appeal to be getting along. The woman started stepping back a little, not coming straight home, felling relaxed. She thought everything was well. One day, the woman got home, and the aunt told her she did not trust the caregiver. The woman asked, her aunt, what was wrong, what did the caregiver do. The aunt said, the caregiver was walking through the house looking at things that she had no business looking at. The woman asked, the caregiver what was she looking for, the caregiver told her she was looking for something the aunt wanted. The woman saw nothing wrong with that. She told her aunt, don't be so fussy. About two weeks later the woman was looking for something, and she could not find it. She did not think about it, she said, she would look for it later. Three weeks passed, and everything appeal to be going OK. One day the caregiver called the woman, and said, she could not make it. The woman had to call out of work, she was going through the house, and she noticed, some things was missing, so she started looking all over. She noticed her checkbook was gone. The woman said she was not going to make an accusation, she was going to wait until the caregiver got back the next day. The caregiver did not show up the next day, the woman tried to call her, and she could not get any answer. The woman called her bank, and founded out money was missing. The woman had to call the police. The aunt said, I told you. The woman started out being actively involved, but then she stopped, she did not listen to her aunt, she did not check the person out, she did not have any important information on the person, she gave the caregiver total control.

Remember, this is how you give someone total control, not listening, not checking, not monitoring/watching, not asking question, and not making yourself visible. This can make the caregiver feel like he/she is running everything, and he/she can do what they want. This confirm things, if you only see your caregiver when, you pay them. Listen to your family member some things may, or may not be true, but if you don't check it out, you will not know. You also send the message to the caregiver, you don't believe what your family member says. You walk around and do not pay attention to anything. You give the caregiver free reign, you do not monitor anything they do. You do not ask the caregiver any questions, even if you see something that doesn't look right. You can see it is very easy to lose your control over things, and you don't have to try hard.

CAREGIVING APPLICATION

FOR THE PERSONAL LEVEL

NAME AND ADDRESS
_____
_____

TELEPHONE NUMBER _____

SOCIAL SECURITY MUMBER (OPTIONAL)_____

DO YOU HAVE A DRIVER LICENSE: YES___ NO___ WHAT STATE AND THE NUMBER

HAVE YOU HAD ANY MOVING VIOLATION YES___ NO___, IF YES EXPLAIN _____
_____

HAVE YOU EVERY BEEN INVOLVE IN AN ALLENGATION OF ABUSE OR NEGLECT YES____ NO____, IF YES EXPLAIN
_____
_____
_____

HAVE YOU BEEN CONVICTED OF, OR ENTERED A PLEA OF GUILTY, NO CONTEST TO A CHARGR OF DOMETIC VIOLENT, ABUSE, NEGLECT. YES____ NO___ IF YES EXPLAINE _____
_____
_____

HOURS OF AVAILABLETY

FULL TIME: 7A-3P_____, 3P-11P_____, 11P-7A_____

PART TIME: LESS THAN 8 HOURS A DAY OR LESS THAN 21 HOURS A WEEK ____

DAYS	Monday	Tuesday	Wednesday	Thursday	Friday	Saturday	Sunday
TIMES							
HOURS							
TOTAL							

(2) JOB EXPERIENCE: NAME, ADDRESS, TITLE, DUTIES, DATES

1. NAME_____
ADRESS_____
_____
TITLE_____
DATES_____
DUTIES_____
_____
_____
_____

2. NAME_____
ADRESS _____
_____
TITLE_____
DATES_____
DUTIES_____
_____
_____
_____

PERSONAL EXPERENCE: RELATIONSHIP, DUTIES, AND DATES (FAMILY, FRIEND, OR ACQUICANT)

1. RELATIONSHIP _____
   DATES _____
   DUTIES _____
   _____
   _____
   _____

WHY DID YOU STOP (DEATH, NOT NEEDED ANYMORE)?
_____

2. RELATIONSHIP _____
   DATES _____
   DUTIES _____
   _____
   _____
   _____

WHY DID YOU STOP, (DEATH, NOT NEEDED ANYMORE)?
_____

(2) JOB REFERENCE: NAME, ADDRESS, PHONE NUMBER, TITLE
1. _____
_____
_____
_____

2 _____
_____
_____
_____

2 PERSONAL LETTER REFERENCE: NAME, DATE

A letter from two people stating you took care of the person, one can be a family member, but the other should be from someone else a friend or neighbor (their name and number).
I_____ KNOW A BACKGROUND CHECK WILL BE DONE.
SIGN,_____

STRESS AND BURNOUT

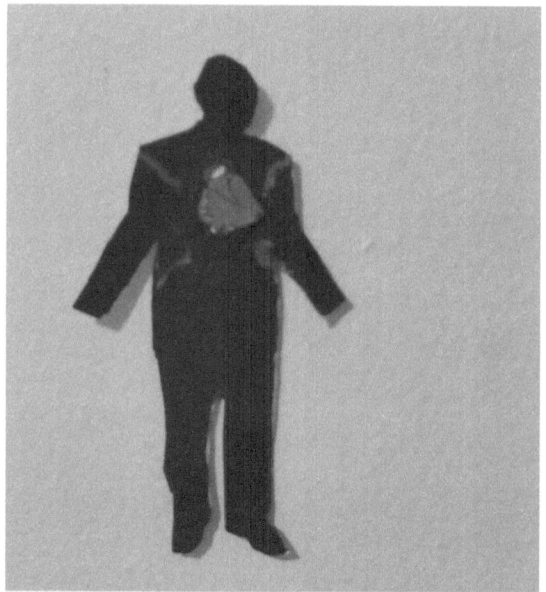

The other things that can affect how you care for someone is called stress, and burnout. I was familiar with these terms, but you don't get the full understanding until you go through it. I use to hear caregivers say, they were stressed, and burned out. I thought they did not know what they were talking about; they looked fine, and they were still working. Later, I found myself in the same condition, stressed out, and burned-out. When I found myself in this situation, I was upset. I thought I was beyond that, because I was a good caregiver. I had been doing this for a long time, and nothing ever affected the way I did my job. I found out no matter what I knew, and how much education I had I was not immune to stress or getting burned-out.

Let me tell you how, I learned, about stress, and burn-out. I had a mild stork, what a wakeup call. First, I want to share some information before I had the stork, and why it took me by surprise. You have read I have been a caregiver for a long time. When I first get out of school, I went to work in a Mental Health Hospital, as a mental health technician, which is a caregiver for that population. I worked around a lot of psychiatrists. One day a group of us were standing in the nursing station. A nurse said "I am so burned out, I do not know, when I had time off beyond my regular days". The director of the unit was standing there, he was a psychiatrist. He gave us some advice. He explained how stressful this field was, and it was easy to get burned out even for him. He decided to give us his secret. Every three months he takes time off. He usually takes a week or more, but if you cannot take a week take three extra days off. If possible, combine them with your regular days off. Do something you like either take a short trip, or just rest. Give your mind, and body a rest from your employer. Every three months repeat the cycle. A lot of us probably do something like this, we just don't realize it, and we do not take the time to regroup we get involved in other stuff instead of resting, and relaxing. I, was intrigued by what he said. I decided to put it to the test. Every three months I would take extra days off combine them with my regular days off. I must admit it worked for years. At one point, I was in a situation where I could not take time off.

I worked as a caregiver, and I evened up being the caregiver for both of my parents at the same time. I was working on the night shift, and coming home, and taking care of my parents doing the day. My mother was bedridden by then, and my father had dementia. My mother had a nurse that came in three days a week for a few hours to help me out. The rest of the week I was on my own, with some family help occasionally. My mother needed wound care daily. Mostly everything had to be done for my mother. She could communicate, she could feed herself, and she was still in her correct state of mind. That was a great help, because I could talk to her. My father needed assistance with his personal care, physical care, and I had very little help with him. My father was confused, he did not know when, or if he had eaten. He could not remember how to use the bathroom. Sometimes he forgot how to walk, I would find him holding onto the wall trying to walk down the hall, and then he would fall. I had to have an alarm system put on the door to keep him from going out. At the end, he could not remember how to swallow his food. I was running around like a machine. I knew I was tired I knew I wasn't getting a lot of sleep. I felt all I had to do was change my batteries, and keep going. I was a caregiver, and I had care for many people at the same time. I could handle things. Well, I could not!

My health started going downhill, and I could not understand why, or what was going on. I knew, I was not getting much sleep, but I did not think that would affect everything. I started losing weight. My appetite had changed. I was not hungry. My hair start to come out, it was coming out in spots. I was feeling very sick. I went to see my doctor, to found out what was wrong. She did some blood work. Some of my levels came back low, and my blood pressure was high. I also had an infection. My blood pressure was high enough, for her to put me on some pills. She treated my infection, but I still felt very sick. She was concerned about my hair coming out. She referred me to a hematologist, and a dermatologist. I was getting afraid, I thought I may have cancer. I saw the dermatologist first, and when she asked me what was going on, I just broke down in tears. I could not explain, what come over me. I told her everything that was going on with my parents. She said, it sounded like I was stressed, and burned out. I did not think that was it. It sounded to sample. I did not think stress could make you sick, I just though it meant you was tied, and you need to sleep. I saw the hematologist, and he wanted to run some more tests. All my test came back fine. He sat me down, and said he thought my problem was stress related. He gave me some lecture on stress, he said I need to get it under control. He also said, looking at things it appeared I was burned out. He recommended I get rid of the stress in my life. He told me I should think about putting my parents in a nursing home, for my health, and theirs, or stop working for a while. I went home, and read the lecture, after reading, and going over my situation, I realize he could be right. I thought about what he said, for a minute, I knew I could not put my parents in a nursing home. I was considering not working for a while. Money was tight, and I could not figure out, how I could do that. I got to the point, I did not care, because my parents were not going into a nursing home. I decided I would work part time. The doctor basically said I would have to do something, or I may not be around to help anyone. He told me I needed to learn stress management.

 I went on the Internet, and looked up stress, and burnout. One site listed some symptoms to look for. To my amazement, I had over half of the symptoms. I then realized, I really was suffering from stress, and burnout. I went to another sight to find out how to manager it. They had a lot of information from, how to reduce stress to overcoming stress. Since I decided to work part time; I could start managing my stress, and get some rest. I also knew, if I did not do something; I could cause harm to my parents, not realizing what I was doing. Then, I remember my pastor teaching. He would tell us to trust in the lord, and he will make the way. He reminded us, God would not put more on us, then we could bear. Those words stuck in my mind so, I kept pushing on. When I made my decision that I was going to put it in the lord's hand, I felt something was lifted. Listen, I was on my way to having a nervous breakdown. I would just start crying for no reason. I felt sick to my stomach. I had headache. I hung in there, my mother died in May, and my father died four months later, September 2007. It was hard, and I thought I had made it. I had done all I could do, and I was at peace.

I took a week off when my mother died, and two weeks off when my father died. I thought that would be all I needed. I went right back to caring for people, not realizing, I did not give myself time to grieve, or rest. Unfortunately, my body had already gone through some changes. Nine months after my father's death, I had a stroke. I wish I could tell you I knew what was happening, and I went to the hospital right way, but I cannot. It is so important to recognize changes in our body, and do not ignore them. My right side was affected, and I could not speak clearly. When I got to the hospital, I understood what people were saying, but I could not respond. I could not do anything but pray, and I was scared. Within two weeks my body starting function almost normal. I had to go too physical therapy for a while. The doctor used words like fortunate, lucky to describe how fast I was getting back to normal. The doctor explained, it could have been worse, but I knew it was god, and I was blessed. They also told me that it came from stress, and high blood pressure. I now have some health issues, I must deal with. I had to make some life changes. I know it can happen again, if I don't manage my stress level, and do what I need to do. I heard about people, and seen people who have had a stork. Some of them recuperated very slow, and some of them had permeant physical damage. Yes, I am blessed. About two months later, I was back at work. I am doing so well, people cannot believe I ever had a stroke. If I, notice any changes in my health, I will seek medical attention right away. I am also trying to get back on that three extra days off plan.

Don't forget stress is something that can sneak up on you, and have you by the throat before you know it. Stress can kill you, and it can break your body down. I encourage everyone who work as a caregiver personal, or professional to learn what stress is, and knows when you are getting burned out. You can become stress any time in your life. Keep a check on your stress level. You should know the symptoms of stress, when working as a caregiver. I did not recognize anything either, I did not know the symptoms. You think you are just tired or exhausted, but things start to get worse. You start to get sick, and don't know why. Education on Stress, and Burnout were the two things I missed as a caregiver. To this day, I get nervous when my blood pressures is high, and it stays that way a couple of days. You should notice changes in your body, but stress, and burn out is hard to pin point. Some of the reason we do not notice we are stress, and burn out are, we need to work, we feel we are the only one that can handle, or do certain things, we ignore our body when it is telling us to rest. I say be careful, and educate yourself about stress, and burned out. No matter what your situation is no one knows everything about everything, but stress can cause you to make bad decisions about yourself, and others.

I heard a story about a woman, who ended up being her husband caregiver. He was dealing with a lot of stress, and he was burned out. Her husband was a teacher for twenty years. Three years ago, he started coming home complaining about the students, and school policies. Things get so bad he made himself sick. He was putting on weigh, and he was not sleeping. He starting getting agitating, and snapping at her, everything at home was getting on his nerves. His wife, convinced him to go to the doctor. The doctor examined him, and asked him some questions about his job, and was he having any problems. Once the doctor finish, and found out what was going on with him, he told him he was under a lot of stress, and he needed to get rid of it. The doctor told him to slow down before things get worse. Her husband felt, if that was all it was he would be ok. A month later, her husband came home, and said, he was having pain in his chest. He refused to go to the hospital, a few minutes later he collapsed on the floor. The ambulance was called, and he was transported to the hospital. It was said, he had a heart attack. Her husband is unable to work now, and he is on a lot of medication. She said, he was depressed now. The doctor made several references to the stress he was experiencing.

A Training Program

A good training program can give you both education, and training, if it is set up right. I got a chance to speak with someone about their training program. This was a big facility, and it was under all the rules, and regulations for a license facility. She took the time to tell me about their training program. They would potentially hire a group of people, but before they went to work on their own, they had to complete this training program. In this class, there were twenty people. The training lasted two weeks 8 hours a day. The director will talk about rules, and regulations. Someone came from adult protective service to talk about abuse, and neglect. Someone went over the operation of the facility, which included emergency procedures, and the layout of the facility. They talked about the type of people they would be working with, and the responsibilities, or duties of the staff. They talked about additional training (CPR). This training program included a lot of information, and you also had a chance to ask questions. This type of training program, might get rid of people who don't really want to do this kind of work. She told me twelve of the people, stayed to become real employees, it doesn't mean all twelve were good caregivers. Some of them, just need a job. Who knows! They completed the training program, which gave them education, and training, some of them probably had the desire. It may cost some money to have a training program, but think how much money you save when you can find good employees; those who want to work in this field for whatever reason. I understand every facility cannot afford to have a big training program, but they can develop a small one. It doesn't matter how long the training program is, it can be a two to three-day program. It is the responsibility of the care facility to provide training for staff. When developing a training program, include things that are important to your facility. You should not give your staff a piece of paper and tell them, "read this, and sign, that you read it". When you sign, something it doesn't always mean you understood it? I found out most people understand what they read, but they do not know how to apply it. For example, you read everyone who lives in a care facility has rights (Two people want to watch a program on TV, but each want to watch a different program that comes on at the same time). They both have the right to watch TV. How do you give both, their rights? It is one thing to say I understood what I read. Do you understand what it means or how it works?

Here are some things you should consider when you developing your training program.

1. Who are the individuals they will be working with (the type of facility, do not give individuals names)?
2. Where are the rules, and regulations handbook kept?
3. Where do you found employees job description?
4. Who do you report information to?
5. Make sure your staff understands the type of work, that is required of them.
6. Documentation training
7. Make sure your staff understand about the hours (there may be overtime that is required, or no overtime ever).
8. Include some role playing (I found that helps a lot when you are trying to explain things).
9. The training program should include information about individual's rights, behavior problems, and information on abuse and neglect.

10. All staff should know the meaning of important words, that is associated with caregivers.
11. Training on diversity. (You should be able to work with all types of people).
12. Talk about communications skills (not having good communication skills can lead to behavior problem, illness going untreated. It also can lead to employee too employee conflicts. and working relationships.
13. How the facility want things done (policies and procedure)?
14. What is the layout of the facility (emergency exit)?
15. Training should include emergency procedure, and none emergency, which could include medical care. Most facilities offer mandatory yearly training for emergency (what to do in cases of a fire). They should provide other yearly training. Make sure you review all of them.

I am sure, you can come up with a lot of other things that may improve the operation of your care facility. I have outlined what I called a basic training program that may help, when you develop yours. Remember, how many days the training program last is not important, it is the information that is important. The information is what is going to get the job done.

A Basic Training Program Outline

Introduction

This is just a basic training program outline to help you develop your own. This outline may not cover all you need for your care facility. It may not be the right outline for your type of care facility. Your care facility may require more information. A training program does not mean you will not have problems in your care facility. My hope, it will cut down on staff turnover, or eliminate the wrong people, before they start working. This will also save you money. I think, it would cut down on abuse and neglect, if people understand what they are doing. It is hard to work in a care facility, and not understand your role or job. A training program gives staff some education. Hopefully, after the training program you end up with people who really want the job (desire). They will continue their education, training, and gain experience.

BASIC TRAINING OUTLINE

I. Identify your facility
   A. What type of facility is this?
   B. Value and mission statement (if you have one)

II. Who are the individuals/clients you will be serving?
   A. Elderly, Alzheimer's, developmental disabilities, and others
   B. What are some of the problems (if any)?
      1. Violent
      2. Confused
      3. Uncooperative
      4. Abusive and aggressive
      5. Ambulatory or not
      6. Communication (yes or no)
   C. Individuals needing special care
      1. Seizures
      2. Alzheimer's/Dementia (wandering)
      3. Prone to falling
      4. Problems eating
      5. Medical problem (special diet)
      6. Incontinent
      7. Behaviors

You may need to bring someone in to help with this part (nurse, behavior specialist, or a physical therapist); it depends on the individual and the facility.

III. Duties
   A. The provider/ facility
   B. Staff
   C. Job description

IV. Procedure for reporting abuse and neglect (complete overview)

V. Individuals rights (complete overview)
VI. Common communication skills, and why it is so important
   1. Facial expression
   2. Body language
   3. Pointing to things
   4. Writing or drawing
   5. Develop your own
VII. Medication and Medical Records, all procedures, and consents (if applies to your facility)
VIII. Incident reporting and procedures
   A. Reportable incidents
   B. Incident writing
IX. Emergency procedure or Manual
   1. Fire, evacuation, disaster (drills)
   2. Emergency exits (layout)
   3. Universal Precaution
   4. CPR and behavior management (if applicable)
X. Employee policies and procedures, rules, and regulations
   A. Code ethics
   B. Adverse weather
   C. Employees Complaints
   D. Cultural awareness
   E. Training
   F. Timesheets
   G. Dressed code
   H. Vacation
   I. Calling in (sick or late)
   J. Holidays
   K. Maintaining confidentiality (no what information you can give out)
XI. Managing facility equipment
   A. Requirement
   B. Computer use (if applicable)
   C. Telephone use (making calls)
   D. Vehicle use (if applicable)

XII. When to call 911
    A. All life-threatening situation (stork, heart attack, etc.)
    B. Any heavy bleeding from an open wound.
XIII. When too informed your supervisor
    1. All life-threatening situation
    2. Accidents
    3. Signs of abuse and neglect
    4. Death
    5. Suddenly illness
    6. Natural disasters
    7. Seizures
    8. Equipment damage
    9. Maintenance problems
    10. Safety problems
    11. Strange behaviors
    12. Violent behaviors
    13. Any other problems related to your resident or the facility.
XIV. How to document
    A. Words to avoid
    B. Phrases to avoid
    C. Practice documentation (give examples)
    D. Definition of words
XV. List of do's and don'ts
XVI. Yearly training (list)
XVII. Misconception about the individual being served (if needed)
XVIII. Location of things
    1. Emergency equipment
    2. Medical equipment
XIX. Questions
XX. Other important information about your agency
XXI. Signature page and date of completion

My hope for this book is:

1. Help caregivers now.
2. Help prepare new caregivers.
3. Get facilities to take notice, and be responsible for their residents.
4. Help start training programs.
5. Stop the abuse, and neglect that are associated with care facilities.
6. Make people realize how important caregivers are.

There are many people who has some experience in caregiving. Most of them do not have a degree, or a title, but with or without a degree, or a title, people are finding themselves in caregiving situations. When I think about some good caregivers in history, with titles, I think about Mother Teresa, and Florence nightingale. They were exceptional caregivers. Some of the things they did was amazing. I cannot say I am one of them, or as good as they were, but being a caregiver has brought out the best in me. It is rewarding, if you really want to be a caregiver, the look on people's faces when you do somethings for them, that they could not do. I have been tested in many ways. My personal life was tested, when I had to take care of my parents. My professional life was tested, staying professional in the work place; when things did not look right, and not being respected. My trustfulness has been tested, followed all the rules and regulations. My spiritual life has been tested, treating people right or the way I would want to be treated. My feelings, emotions, toward the people I was caring for has been tested. My sanity has been tested, trying to figure out why people was doing some of the thing they were doing to their clients/residents. My personality has been tested, what was I made of? My strength has been tested; how long can I be a caregiver. Remember, it is not always the facility fault, some people no they should not be a caregiver. Even with all the information out there you just can't catch all the bad caregivers some of them get away.

THE END

THIS BOOK IS DEDICATED TO THE
MEMORY OF MY PARENTS

ANNIE B. HARRIS
EARLEY HARRIS SR

INDEX

A

abuse, 27–28, 31, 35, 71

B

burnout, 11, 106, 109, 111

C

care facility, questions to ask before working in, 39
caregiver, 20, 23
   daily living skills assisted by, 50
   dos and don'ts for, 51
   reasons to work as, 33
   tips before hiring someone as, 93
   work as, 9, 14, 29, 33–35, 39, 52–53, 55

D

desire, 10, 65–72, 113, 116
dignity, 24
documentation, 54, 61

E

education, 67, 71

H

Harris, Carrie
   experience with care facilities, 84
   health concern, 110
   lessons learned while working as caregiver, 28
   observations as caregiver, 35
human service worker. *See* caregiver

I

intellectual disability, 53
   problems dealing with people having, 52

J

John (caregiver), 97–100

L

language game. *See* documentation

N

neglect, 27–35, 71

R

respect, 23–24

S

stress, 109–11

www.ingramcontent.com/pod-product-compliance
Lightning Source LLC
Chambersburg PA
CBHW022013170526
45157CB00003B/1229